SOUPiNG

Alison Velázquez

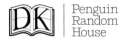

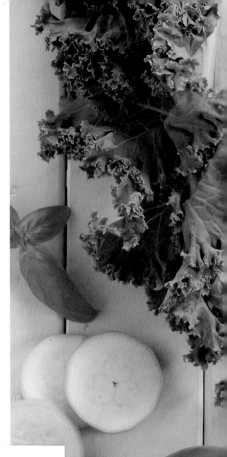

To my family, who have been there from the beginning and believed in me.

Publisher: Mike Sanders
Associate Publisher: Billy Fields
Senior Acquisitions Editor: Brook Farling
Development Editor: Ann Barton
Senior Jacket Creative: Nicola Powling
Book Designer: XAB Design
Photographer: Brian Wetzstein
Food Stylist: Mollie Hayward
Prepress Technician: Brian Massey
Proofreader: Laura Caddell
Indexer: Heather McNeill

First American Edition, 2015
Published in the United States by DK Publishing
6081 E. 82nd Street, Indianapolis, Indiana 46250

ISBN: 978-1-46544-930-6
Library of Congress Catalog Card Number: 2015941799

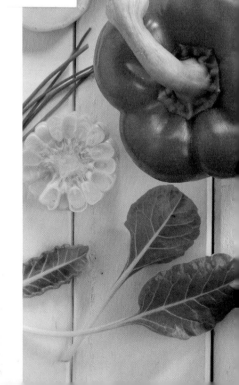

33614056477234

Note: This publication contains the opinions and ideas of its author(s). It is intended to
provide helpful and informative material on the subject matter covered. It is sold with
the understanding that the author(s) and publisher are not engaged in rendering
professional services in the book. If the reader requires personal assistance or advice,
a competent professional should be consulted. The author(s) and publisher specifically
disclaim any responsibility for any liability, loss, or risk, personal or otherwise, which is
incurred as a consequence, directly or indirectly, of the use and application of any of
the contents of this book.

Trademarks: All terms mentioned in this book that are known to be or are suspected
of being trademarks or service marks have been appropriately capitalized. Alpha Books,
DK, and Penguin Random House LLC cannot attest to the accuracy of this information.
Use of a term in this book should not be regarded as affecting the validity of any
trademark or service mark.

DK books are available at special discounts when purchased in bulk for sales
promotions, premiums, fund-raising, or educational use. For details, contact: DK
Publishing Special Markets, 345 Hudson Street, New York, New York 10014 or
SpecialSales@dk.com.

For further information see: www.dkimages.com
www.dk.com

A WORLD OF IDEAS:
SEE ALL THERE IS TO KNOW

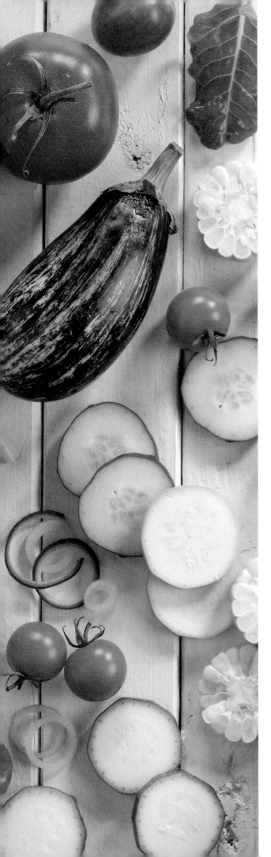

CONTENTS

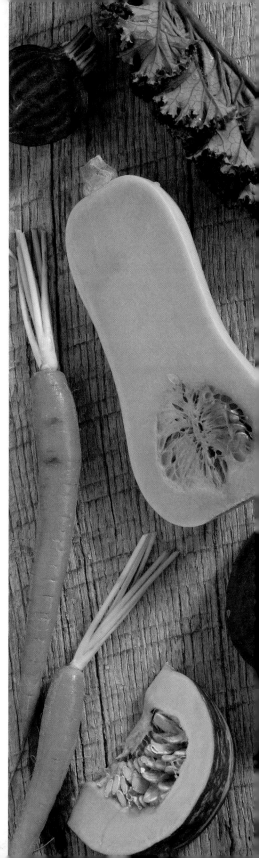

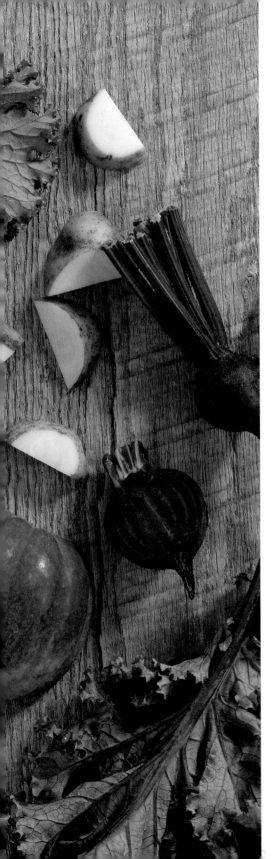

INTRODUCTION

Soup is as old as the history of cooking. Simmering simple ingredients to make nutritious and filling meals has been practiced for centuries.

Be it gazpacho, vischyssoise, corn chowder, or tortilla soup, all are variations on the same theme that have been influenced and shaped by local ingredients and traditions. In the past, there was nothing trendy about soup; it was just nutrition-based eating.

Kale, quinoa, and fresh-pressed juices have all had their moments in the spotlight. Now is the time for soup. However, I'm not talking about shelf stable, preservative-filled canned soups, or cream-and-butter-rich restaurant soups. I'm talking about back to basics—to what soups were and should be. Fresh, preservative-free vegetable soups that are full of nutrients and brimming with bright flavors.

The intent of this book is not only to offer a fresh take on what soup can be, but to introduce soup as a lifestyle known as "souping." Souping can simply be the idea of integrating fresh, nutrient-dense soups into your daily diet to provide additional nutrition and hydration. Or, for those looking for further benefits like detoxification and alkalinity, souping can mean sticking to a diet of these nutrient-rich soup blends for a set amount of time as a cleanse program.

This collection of over 75 hot and chilled soup recipes, along with 10 different cleanse programs, aims to make souping at home easy. These carefully crafted recipes are meant to provide the right mix of nutrition, variety, and deliciousness. Souping is an easy, convenient, and delicious way to hydrate, nourish, and energize the body. You shouldn't have to go to extremes to feel the benefits of mindful eating. I am excited to share some of my favorite health blends and hope that these recipes help make eating healthy at home a little bit simpler.

Just heat, sip, enjoy, and repeat.

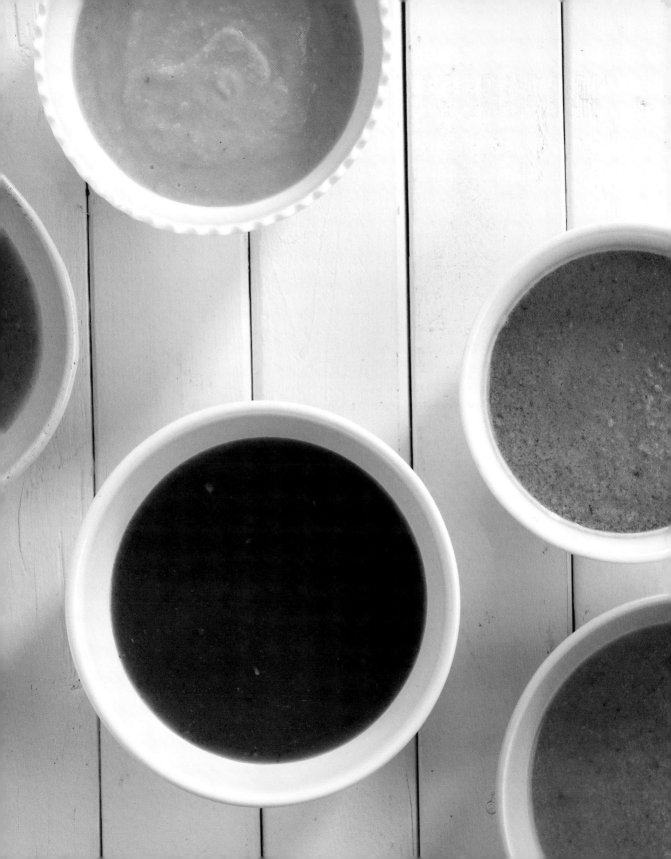

1
SOUPING ESSENTIALS

In this part, you'll learn what souping is and why you should be making it part of your healthy lifestyle. You'll get ideas for stocking your pantry with essential ingredients, tips on selecting kitchen equipment, and suggestions for storing your soups in order to make souping as easy as possible.

WHAT IS SOUPING?

Souping is the idea of incorporating nutrient-dense, vegetable-based soups into your diet. Whether you embark on an all-soup cleanse or just replace one or two meals a day with soup, it's an ideal way to pump your body full of nutrients, antioxidants, and phytochemicals.

BENEFITS OF A SOUP CLEANSE

Soups are a great way to build more healthy and satisfying meals into your diet. Because soups are high in water and fiber, but low in sugar, they are filling without causing spikes in blood sugar.

The mind-body benefits of a soup cleanse are many:
★ flushes out harmful toxins
★ encourages weight loss
★ boosts immunity
★ increases energy
★ reduces cravings
★ aids digestion
★ improves gut health
★ refocuses the mind
★ eases headaches
★ brightens the skin

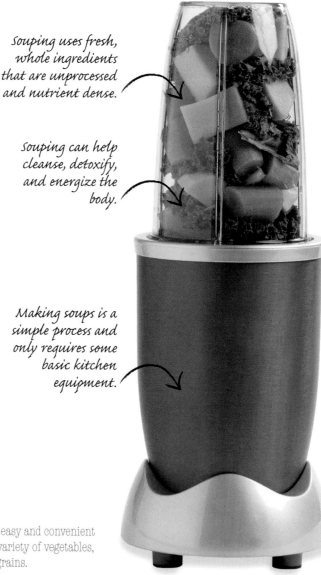

Souping uses fresh, whole ingredients that are unprocessed and nutrient dense.

Souping can help cleanse, detoxify, and energize the body.

Making soups is a simple process and only requires some basic kitchen equipment.

Souping offers an easy and convenient way to eat a wide variety of vegetables, fruits, and whole grains.

SOUPING VS. JUICING

You may be wondering how souping compares to another popular diet trend, juicing. While juices are extracted from fruits and vegetables, leaving the fibrous pulp behind, soups are made by puréeing whole ingredients, and they retain beneficial fiber. Souping and juicing share many positive attributes, but souping is more versatile and has added health benefts, thanks to the increased fiber, fat, and protein, and fewer sweet ingredients.

SOUPING

nutrient-dense, vegetable-based soups

✓ Easily adaptable for diet and allergy restrictions

✓ Hydrating

✓ Low in fat and calories

✓ Easy to digest

✓ Filling and high in fiber

✓ Low in sugar (no blood sugar spikes)

✓ Includes protein from legumes, greens, and grains

✓ Includes healthy fats, such as coconut oil and olive oil

✓ Can be served hot or cold

✓ Variety of flavors, from savory to sweet

✓ Can be made ahead and frozen

JUICING

raw juice made from fruits and vegetables

✓ Vegan and gluten free

✓ Hydrating

✓ Low in fat and calories

✓ Easy to digest

✓ Energizing

✗ Low in fiber

✗ May be high in sugar (natural fructose)

✗ Not a good source of protein or healthy fats

✗ Primarily served chilled

✗ Usually sweet, with few savory options

✗ Short shelf life

✗ Less economical due to the volume of ingredients required

HEALTH BENEFITS OF SOUPING

A soup cleanse provides both physical and mental benefits. Wholesome, vegetable-based soups are filling and satisfying, as well as rich in beneficial antioxidants and phytochemicals.

A FRESH START

Just making the decision to cleanse is a huge step in the right direction. By breaking your normal routine, you have a definitive starting point, as well as motivation to continue with healthy habits. A cleanse provides a set amount of time to reset and prioritize your goals going forward. By changing your diet in a focused, specific way, you become more mindful of your eating.

Detoxification
You are constantly exposed to environmental toxins. A cleanse helps flush these toxins from your body.

Weight Loss
Lifestyle and diet directly affect your weight. A calorie-controlled cleanse brings you back to basics and can help drop pounds while curbing cravings.

BODY BENEFITS

Improved Gut Health
Fiber and nutrient rich, a cleanse can help promote proper digestion and restore gut health.

Hydration
The body functions best with proper hydration. A cleanse dictates a schedule that will boost your body's hydration.

FOCUS ON NUTRITION

While you cleanse, you avoid foods that may be detrimental to your physical and mental well-being, such as refined carbohydrates, sugar, and caffeine. Instead, a soup cleanse relies on wholesome, nutrient-rich ingredients that deliver the sustenance you need. Even two or three days of souping can make a difference to your physical and mental health. Incorporating soups and soup cleanses into your diet on a regular basis can result in lasting benefits.

MIND BENEFITS

Improved Mood
Diet choices can affect your metabolism, hormones, and neurotransmitters, which in turn affect your emotions. A vegetable-rich cleanse that is low in sugar keeps these variables in check.

Increased Mental Clarity
Poor nutrition can lead to mental fogginess and lethargy. Both hydrating and nourishing, a cleanse can reawaken the senses.

Better Sleep
Poor nutrition and dehydration can affect the quality of your sleep. A cleanse can be restorative for the body and encourage regular sleep patterns.

Reduced Cravings
Cutting out sugar and processed foods through a cleanse allows you to reset your body. Withdrawal will only last a few days, after which your cravings will subside.

Fewer Headaches
Fatigue and poor hydration can lead to headaches. A cleanse restores proper hydration and nutrition.

ESSENTIAL INGREDIENTS

Healthy and delicious soups start with high-quality, nutrient-rich ingredients. Seek out organic, seasonal produce when possible, and stock up on key dry goods such as oils, spices, and legumes.

INGREDIENT Q&A

Q What kind of salt should I use?
A Look for mineral-rich, unrefined salts, such as sea salt. Avoid table salt, which is highly refined.

Q Is it okay to substitute dried herbs for fresh herbs?
A Dried herbs can be substituted for fresh herbs in cooked soups. Because dried herbs are more potent than fresh, reduce the amount by two-thirds. Avoid using dried herbs in soups that are raw or chilled.

Q Can I use store-bought broths?
A Store-bought broths will work in a pinch, but it's highly recommended that you make your own broth. Store-bought broths are often high in sodium and may contain MSG and other additives.

Q What kind of onions should I use?
A In most cases, yellow onions are the best choice. Use sweet onions for a milder flavor and red or white onions for a more pungent flavor.

Q Can I use canned or frozen fruits and vegetables?
A Nothing beats fresh produce, but when fresh isn't available, opt for frozen over canned. When purchasing, make sure there are no added sauces or seasonings.

Q Do I have to use purified water for my soups?
A Purified water has been filtered or processed to remove trace contaminants and impurities, making it an ideal ingredient for soups. Tap water may contain chlorine and other chemicals, which can pose health risks and reduce the health benefits of other ingredients.

Q Where can I get bones to make my bone broth?
A Bones can be found inexpensively at your local butcher shop, or you can save the bones after roasting a chicken or cooking bone-in cuts of meat. Wrap the bones in foil, place in a freezer bag, and freeze until ready to use.

PANTRY

Many of the soups in this book rely on a few key ingredients. Keeping your pantry stocked with these staples will make it easier to shop for soups.

Spices: Have sea salt and black pepper on hand, as well as other basic spices such as red pepper flakes, cumin, and chili powder. Store spices in tightly closed containers, away from light.

Oils: Coconut oil and olive oil are used to cook vegetables for soups. Look for cold-pressed, virgin (or extra-virgin) varieties.

Garlic: Fresh garlic should be stored in the pantry, not the refrigerator. Keep garlic bulbs loose, with airflow to prevent decay.

Onions: Onions add savory flavor and mouth-watering aroma to many soups. Like garlic, onions are best stored in the dark, at room temperature, with plenty of airflow.

Grains: Look for less-familiar ancient grains such as quinoa, freekeh, amaranth, and millet, which contain more protein and nutrients than white or even brown rice.

Legumes: Beans are a great way to add protein and body to soups. Keep a supply of canned or dried chickpeas and black beans on hand, as well as dried lentils.

Canned diced tomatoes: Canned diced tomatoes (regular or fire-roasted) are packaged at the peak of ripeness and deliver rich umami flavor as well as lycopene. Look for low-sodium varieties.

Light coconut milk: Coconut milk is shelf-stable and brings creaminess and body to both sweet and savory soups without added dairy.

Nuts: Cashews and almonds can be soaked and blended to deliver protein and creamy texture to soups. Use raw, unsalted varieties.

Purified water: Water is an essential ingredient in soup making, and the type you use can make a difference. Keep a stock of purified water to get the most nutrients from your soups.

FRIDGE & FREEZER

Fresh produce and meats are vital to making delicious, nutrient-rich soups. These are some of the most-often used fresh ingredients in this book.

Carrots: A base for many soups is the classic mirepoix mix of carrots, onions, and celery. Carrots, which are rich in vitamin A, are essential to this trio and add a slight sweetness to balance out the flavors.

Celery: Another crucial ingredient to the mirepoix mix is celery. Celery adds an aromatic note, which delivers depth and complexity of flavor.

Spinach: Iron-rich spinach has a mild flavor, which complements both sweet and savory soups. Look for baby spinach, which is slightly sweeter with tender leaves.

Fresh herbs: Herbs introduce lots of flavor and freshness to your soups with no additional calories. Keep fresh basil, parsley, and cilantro on hand.

Fresh ginger and turmeric: Fresh ginger and turmeric are inexpensive and will keep a long time. These fresh spices are nutritional powerhouses that complement a range of dishes, from savory to sweet.

Lemons: A great source of vitamin C, a squeeze of lemon can boost the nutritional content and brighten the overall flavor profile of a soup.

Chiles: Chile peppers are a great way to add flavor without calories. Try poblano, jalapeño, and serrano peppers.

Coconut water: Hydrating coconut water replenishes electrolytes and makes a great base for chilled soups.

Bone-in chicken pieces and other meat bones: Animal bones are the foundation of nutrient-rich bone broths.

Homemade broths: Broth freezes well, so make a big batch when you have time and freeze it in small containers for later use.

MAKING SOUPS

One of the best things about souping is that most of the recipes come together quickly and can be prepared in advance, making it a manageable diet that doesn't require spending every evening at the stove.

TYPES OF SOUPS

Almost all of the soups in this book are puréed or strained for a smooth texture and ease of sipping on the go. Soups may be served hot or cold.

Hot Soups

Soups that are meant to be served warm or hot are typically prepared by cooking ingredients, either on the stovetop or roasting, and then puréeing them along with the cooking liquid.

Chilled Soups

Chilled soups may be prepared from cooked or raw ingredients. Soups that do not freeze well are often those made with raw ingredients, such as banana or melon. When making a chilled soup, be sure to allow time for refrigeration.

Broths and Consommés

These clear, thin liquids are prepared by simmering vegetables and/or meat or poultry bones in water for an extended time, allowing the beneficial minerals to be drawn out. Broths and consommés often include aromatics, such as ginger, for added flavor and nutrients. Broths are simply strained before using, while consommés are clarified to remove impurities, usually by using egg whites.

TOOLS AND EQUIPMENT

Soups don't require a lot of special kitchen equipment. In addition to a blender, you'll need the following:

★ Baking sheet
★ Chef's knife
★ Cutting board
★ Ladle
★ Mesh seive
★ Paring knife
★ Peeler
★ Prep bowls
★ Skillet
★ Spatula
★ Stockpot or Dutch oven
★ Wooden spoon

Hot Stuff

When a recipe calls for blending hot soups, take care. The steam from the hot ingredients creates pressure that can push the lid right off the blender, splashing liquid everywhere (including on you). If you're using a regular blender, remove the center plug from the lid and cover it with a folded dish towel while blending to prevent steam buildup. Another option is using an immersion blender. Take the cooking pot off the heat and carefully purée the ingredients in the pot.

1 PREP

A crucial aspect of souping success is allowing enough time to plan and prepare. Once you have selected a cleanse, create a master list of all the ingredients you will need for the cleanse, and shop for ingredients ahead of time. Keeping your kitchen stocked with staples will cut down on shopping time.

2 COOK AND BLEND

To make cooking manageable, it's recommended that you begin preparing soups a week ahead of your cleanse. When you are ready to cook, make sure you have the ingredients for all the soups you are making that day, along with your basic utensils. Start by prepping all the ingredients, like mincing garlic and dicing onion. Once all your ingredients are prepped, the actual cooking goes quickly.

BLENDER

A traditional blender is capable of puréeing large quantities of soup, and is able to achieve a smooth consistency, even for tough or fibrous ingredients. For the smoothest and easiest blending, you may consider investing in a high-powered blender.

IMMERSION BLENDER

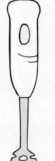

A handheld immersion blender allows you to purée soups right in the pot that you used for cooking. Immersion blenders are great for safely puréeing hot ingredients, and they also cut down on dishes to wash.

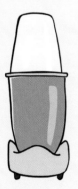

BULLET STYLE BLENDER

A bullet-style blender is useful for making single servings of soups, especially those with perishable ingredients. It's also simple to clean.

FOOD PROCESSOR

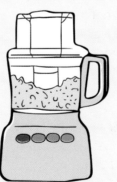

A food processor can be used in place of a blender if needed, but it may not achieve as smooth a texture and transferring liquid ingredients to and from the bowl may be difficult.

3 STORE

If you're not eating your soup immediately, transfer it to an airtight container and store in the refrigerator or freezer (if the soup can be frozen). Most soups can be refrigerated for several days or frozen for up to eight weeks. To defrost frozen soups, allow them to thaw for 24 hours in the refrigerator. Before serving, you may want to blend your soups briefly to recombine ingredients.

STORING SOUPS

Most soups can be prepared days or even weeks in advance, provided you store them properly. Cook in batches, and invest in a set of freezer-safe, single-serving containers for portioning and storing your soups.

COOK IN BATCHES

It takes almost the same amount of time to prepare a single batch of soup as it does to make several batches of that same soup. Save time and energy by making double or triple batches. In most cases, extra portions can be frozen for a later date. Check the storage information on the recipe for refrigeration and freezing times.

STORE IN SINGLE-SERVING PORTIONS

Rather than ladling out one serving at a time from a large container, immediately portion your soups into single-serving containers. In addition to cooling more quickly, single-serving containers make efficient use of refrigerator and freezer space, are easy to grab and go, and ensure that you consume the intended amount of calories.

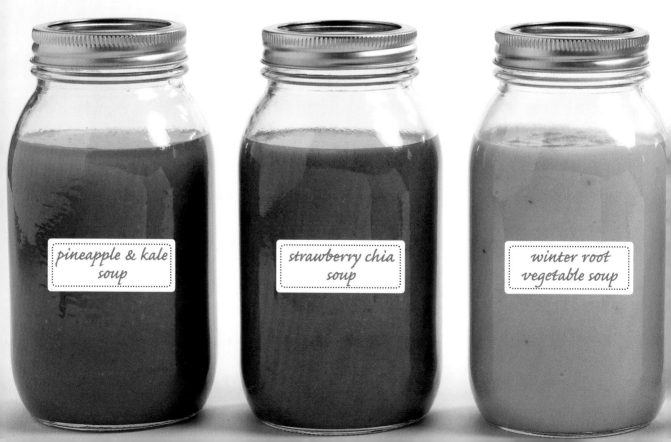

pineapple & kale soup

strawberry chia soup

winter root vegetable soup

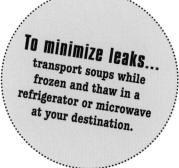

To minimize leaks...
transport soups while frozen and thaw in a refrigerator or microwave at your destination.

CHOOSE THE RIGHT CONTAINER

Look for airtight, leak-proof containers that can withstand heat, so you can easily microwave your soups on the go. Your containers should be large enough to hold at least two cups of soup, with room to heat and stir. Glass Mason jars or sturdy plastic containers with screw-top lids are great for storing and transporting soups.

10 Soups to Freeze

Most of the recipes in this book freeze well. Make a double batch of one of these freezer-friendly soups to get started.

1 Black Bean Poblano Soup
2 Nutmeg Sweet Potato Soup
3 Broccoli Arugula Soup
4 Zucchini Soup with Basil
5 Curried Butternut Soup
6 French Lentil Soup
7 Winter Root Vegetable Soup
8 Butternut Black Bean Soup
9 Sesame Vegetable Broth
10 Carrot & Fennel Soup

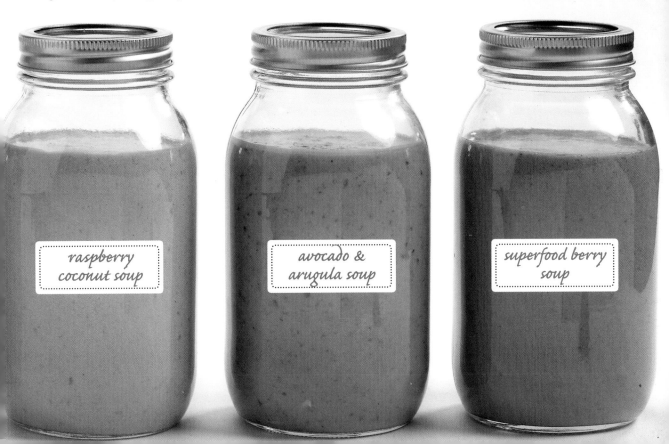

raspberry coconut soup

avocado & arugula soup

superfood berry soup

PREPARING FOR A CLEANSE

This book contains 10 soup cleanses, each of which is designed to support or nourish specific aspects of your health. Choose a cleanse that speaks to your health needs and fits your upcoming schedule.

SELECT A CLEANSE

★ Choose a time to cleanse when you don't have a lot going on in your social or work calendar.

★ Ask a friend or your partner to join you in doing your cleanse. It's always easier when you have someone to hold you accountable.

THE 10 CLEANSES

1 **Metabolism Boost:** Reset and boost metabolism. PAGE 34

2 **Energize:** Boost energy and stamina. PAGE 46

3 **Weight Loss:** Reduce bloating and kick-start weight loss. PAGE 66

4 **Hydrate:** Refresh and hydrate your body. PAGE 78

5 **Alkalize:** Rebalance your body's pH levels. PAGE 98

6 **Beauty Reboot:** Nourish your hair, skin, and nails. PAGE 110

7 **Detoxify:** Remove impurities from your body. PAGE 132

8 **Immune Boost:** Strengthen and boost your immune system. PAGE 144

9 **Digestive Health:** Soothe and restore natural balance to your digestive system. PAGE 164

10 **Anti-Inflammatory:** Reduce inflammation and combat joint pain. PAGE 176

PREPARE FOR A CLEANSE

2 WEEKS BEFORE

★ Select your cleanse.

★ Review the shopping list for your cleanse and purchase any pantry staples or other non-perishable items you need.

1 WEEK BEFORE

★ Make sure you have appropriate storage containers for storing your soups. If you plan to store your soups in individual portions, you will need six 2-cup containers for each day of the cleanse.

★ Purchase ingredients for the two soups that you will make and freeze ahead.

★ Make two soups for your cleanse and freeze them.

4 DAYS BEFORE

★ Purchase the ingredients for your remaining soups as well as healthy foods to begin transitioning your diet as you prepare for your cleanse.

3 DAYS BEFORE

★ In the three days before your cleanse, prepare the remaining four soups.

★ Start transitioning your diet as outlined in your cleanse, weaning yourself off of sugars and processed foods.

CLEANSE Q&A

Q **Do I have to consume the soups in a certain order?**
A No. While there is a suggested order based on the health benefits of specific soups (for example, starting the day with a metabolism-boosting soup), it will not impact the outcome of the cleanse to choose a different order.

Q **Can I exercise while cleansing?**
A Movement and exercise are always good for the body. Just be aware that your caloric intake may be lower than usual, so you may not want to burn too many calories.

Q **How will cleansing make me feel?**
A Everyone's experiences differ based on what their normal diets and habits may be. Most people find the first day to be the most challenging. Some people experience lethargy or headaches. Don't worry; this is just a sign that your body has registered a change. The headaches and tiredness should abate after the first or second day of cleansing.

Q **Can I drink coffee?**
A Coffee is an acidic food that takes your body out of its optimal alkaline state. One of the great benefits of a souping cleanse is that it will help curb cravings. For the short time you cleanse, try to forego coffee. If you really need caffeine, try green tea.

Q **Can I freeze the soups?**
A The majority of the soups in this book can be frozen. Look for freezing instructions in the Storage section of the recipe. (Defrost frozen soups for 24 hours in the refrigerator before serving.)

Q **Can I eat solid foods while cleansing?**
A If you feel the need to chew or eat other foods while cleansing, try raw or steamed veggies with a squeeze of lime, or half an avocado with a sprinkle of sea salt.

Q **Will I lose weight?**
A Whether or not you lose weight depends on what your diet is normally; however, because the cleanses are low in calories, many people do experience weight loss.

Q **Will I be hungry?**
A Most people find that they are not hungry at all; in fact, some people have trouble finishing all their soups in a day. The fiber from the vegetables and the high volume of water make for a very filling combination.

Q **Will cleansing slow my metabolism?**
A A soup cleanse still provides sufficient calories to keep your metabolism moving. Many of the soups include ingredients that may actually speed up your metabolism.

FOLLOWING A CLEANSE

To get the most out of your cleanse, prepare your body by making slight modifications to your diet in the days leading up to and following the cleanse.

Adjusting your diet before and after a cleanse helps to maximize cleanse benefits and prevents you from returning to old habits too quickly. Whether you've curbed a craving, lost weight, gained energy, or simply kick-started a healthier lifestyle, transitioning properly can help keep the momentum going. Even if you only plan to cleanse for a day or two, modifying your diet before and afterward will help to ease the transition. While you're cleansing, stick to your prepared soups and avoid snacking or drinking sweetened beverages.

WHEN SHOULD I CLEANSE?	TRANSITIONING INTO A CLEANSE	DURING THE CLEANSE	TRANSITIONING OUT OF A CLEANSE
When to cleanse is entirely up to you, depending on your lifestyle and your diet. Some people like to cleanse quarterly to reboot the body as the seasons change. Others prefer monthly cleanses. Some people cleanse after a particularly indulgent weekend or vacation. If weight loss is your goal, you may choose to cleanse more frequently over a shorter period of time. There is no right or wrong time to cleanse. Listen to your body. A nutrient-dense, vegetable-based diet is always a smart idea.	**3 Days Before:** Begin removing processed food from your diet and focus on eating whole foods, including vegetables, legumes, lean meats, and grains. **2 Days Before:** Begin removing meat, poultry, and dairy products from your diet. Focus on a vegetable-heavy diet supplemented with fish, grains, and legumes. **1 Day Before:** Remove all animal products from your diet and focus on a vegetable-based diet supplemented with legumes, grains, and nuts. Drink at least 8 cups of water.	★ Try to eat only the soups you've prepared for your cleanse. ★ Drink 1 to 2 cups of water or unsweetened tea between each soup. (Aim for 8 cups of water per day.) ★ Engage in light exercise daily. ★ Sleep for 7 to 8 hours each night.	**1 Day After:** Start with a vegetable-based diet supplemented with legumes, grains, and nuts. Drink at least 8 cups of water. **2 Days After:** Continue to focus on a vegetable-based diet supplemented by grains and legumes. Begin to add fish to your diet, if this is something you'd like to include. Drink at least 8 cups of water. **3 Days After:** Continue to focus on a vegetable-based diet supplemented by grains and legumes. If you'd like to add other lean proteins, like chicken or pork, do so. Drink at least 8 cups of water.

The vegetable- and broth-based soups in this book are designed to keep you full during your cleanse while delivering key nutrients and antioxidants.

Low-sugar, high-volume soups keep you full and curb cravings.

2

SPRING SOUPING

Spring souping features cleanses for boosting your metabolism and energizing your body. The bright flavors of the spring harvest are highlighted in these recipes, which are lighter in texture yet still incredibly satisfying. The minimal ingredients in these soups allow the delicate flavors of spring to shine.

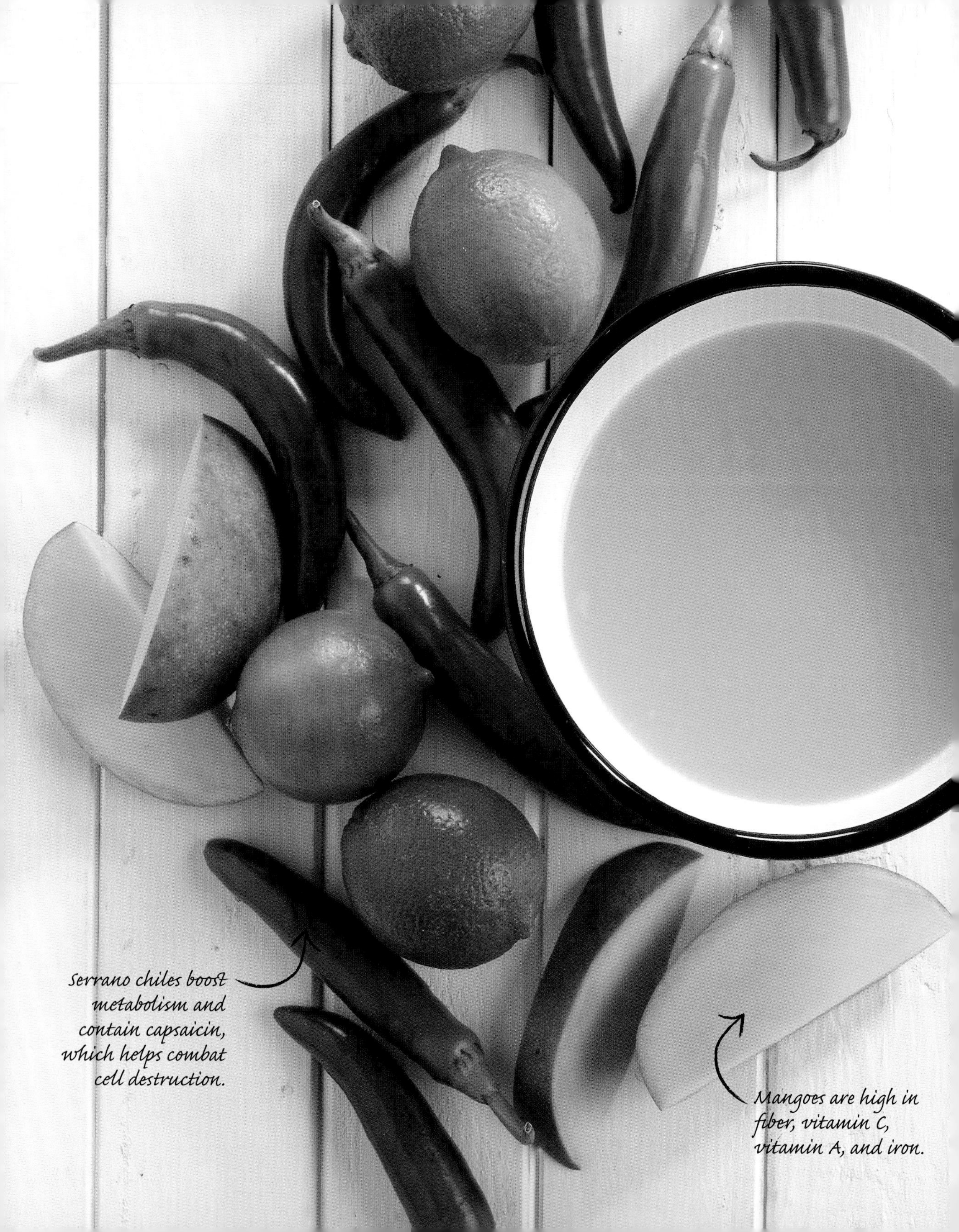

Serrano chiles boost
metabolism and
contain capsaicin,
which helps combat
cell destruction.

Mangoes are high in
fiber, vitamin C,
vitamin A, and iron.

MANGO SOUP WITH LIME

Mangoes give this **light, refreshing elixir** smoothness and body, as well as a **creamy texture**. The sweet mango is balanced by the **tartness of lime juice** and **mild heat of serrano pepper**. Serve chilled.

 PREP & COOK
35 minutes

 QUANTITY
Makes 4 cups
Serving size 2 cups

STORAGE
Refrigerated 5 days
Frozen 8 weeks

INGREDIENTS

2 large mangoes, peeled
  and cubed

¼ serrano pepper, seeds
  removed and minced

Juice of 1 lime

3 cups purified water

METHOD

1 Place mangoes, serrano pepper, lime juice, and water in blender. Purée for 30 seconds or until smooth.

2 Transfer blending vessel to refrigerator for 30 minutes to chill. Blend briefly before serving, if needed.

NUTRITION PER SERVING

calories	214
total fat	2g
cholesterol	0mg
sodium	5mg
carbohydrate	54g
dietary fiber	6g
sugars	47g
protein	3g

To make...
Creamy Mango Soup, add ½ cup Greek yogurt and 1 tsp. fresh grated ginger to the blender.

Cucumber's high water and fiber content make it incredibly hydrating and great for digestion.

AVOCADO & ARUGULA SOUP

With **creamy avocado, spicy arugula,** and **hydrating cucumber,** this refreshing soup has a **smooth, silky texture** highlighted by herbal notes of **fresh basil** and **cilantro.** Serve chilled.

 PREP & COOK
10 minutes

 QUANTITY
Makes 4 cups
Serving size 2 cups

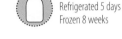 **STORAGE**
Refrigerated 5 days
Frozen 8 weeks

INGREDIENTS

½ avocado, skin and seed removed

2 cups cucumber, peeled and sliced

1 cup baby arugula, tightly packed

1 cup butter lettuce, roughly chopped

¼ cup fresh cilantro, stems removed and minced

2 TB. fresh basil, minced

1½ TB. red wine vinegar

2½ cups purified water

¼ tsp. salt

⅛ tsp. pepper

METHOD

1 Place avocado, cucumber, arugula, butter lettuce, cilantro, basil, red wine vinegar, and water in blender. Purée for 30 seconds or until smooth.

2 If desired, transfer blending vessel to refrigerator for 30 minutes to chill. Season with salt and pepper and blend briefly to recombine ingredients.

NUTRITION PER SERVING

calories	89
total fat	6g
cholesterol	0mg
sodium	303mg
carbohydrate	7g
dietary fiber	4g
sugars	3g
protein	2g

For a spicy kick...
add a pinch of red pepper flakes or 2 tsp. minced serrano pepper to the blender.

Almond milk contains energy-boosting riboflavin and vitamin E, which helps boosts immunity.

Goji berries are high in antioxidants, fiber, and iron.

SUPERFOOD BERRY SOUP

This **sweet and slightly tart** soup is a delicious way to start the day. Creamy Greek yogurt provides a **protein-rich base,** while strawberries and goji berries add a **fruity tang.** Serve chilled.

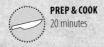 **PREP & COOK**
20 minutes

 QUANTITY
Makes 3 cups
Serving size 2 cups

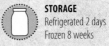 **STORAGE**
Refrigerated 2 days
Frozen 8 weeks

INGREDIENTS

2 TB. ground flax seeds

3 TB. dried goji berries

1 cup unsweetened almond milk

2 cups strawberries, hulled and quartered

½ cup Greek yogurt (2% plain)

2 tsp. vanilla

2 tsp. honey

METHOD

1 In a small bowl, combine ground flax seeds, goji berries, and almond milk. Let sit for 15 minutes to allow goji berries to soften and flax to thicken.

2 Place almond milk mixture, strawberries, Greek yogurt, vanilla, and honey in a blender. Purée for 30 seconds or until smooth.

Top with...
whole flax seeds for a nutty crunch, or use frozen strawberries for a thicker consistency.

NUTRITION PER SERVING

calories	308
total fat	8g
cholesterol	6mg
sodium	218mg
carbohydrate	46g
dietary fiber	8g
sugars	32g
protein	14g

In addition to being high in vitamin C, bell peppers are a good source of vitamin B6, which helps detoxify the liver.

KALE & BELL PEPPER SOUP

This mellow soup blends **mild yellow peppers, smooth avocado,** and **crisp cucumber** with **nutrient-dense kale** for a **refreshingly light** and simple **spring meal.** Serve chilled.

PREP & COOK
20 minutes

QUANTITY
Makes 4 cups
Serving size 2 cups

STORAGE
Refrigerated 5 days
Freezing not recommended

INGREDIENTS

2 cups cucumber, peeled
  and diced

2 cups yellow bell pepper,
  diced

⅔ cup kale, stems removed
  and roughly chopped

⅔ cup celery, diced

½ cup basil, chopped

2 tsp. lemon juice

½ avocado

2 cups purified water

⅛ tsp. salt

⅛ tsp. pepper

METHOD

1 In a blender, combine cucumber, yellow bell pepper, kale, celery, basil, lemon juice, avocado, and water.

2 Purée for 30 seconds or until smooth. Season with salt and pepper and blend briefly to combine.

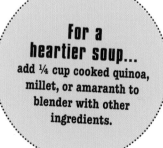

For a heartier soup...
add ¼ cup cooked quinoa, millet, or amaranth to blender with other ingredients.

NUTRITION PER SERVING

calories	154
total fat	8g
cholesterol	0mg
sodium	341mg
carbohydrate	19g
dietary fiber	8g
sugars	9g
protein	4g

METABOLISM BOOSTER
3-DAY CLEANSE

Metabolism is the process the body uses to break down nutrients to produce energy. A healthy metabolism helps to maintain a normal body weight, keep bodily processes functioning, and ward off fatigue. Poor diet choices can directly affect your metabolism. Use this cleanse to reboot and maintain metabolic health.

Follow for 3 days. After your cleanse, try incorporating these metabolism-boosting soups into your daily diet for continued metabolic health.

Shopping List

Fridge/Freezer
Serrano pepper (1)
Poblano pepper (1)
Onions (6 medium)
Carrot (3 medium)
Celery (4 stalks)
Garlic (19 cloves)
Fresh ginger (3 [1 in.; 2.5cm] pieces)
Butternut squash (2 small)
Baby spinach (2 cups)
Mangoes (2)
Limes (9)
Cilantro (1 bunch)
Parsley (5 stems)

Pantry
Olive oil (½ cup)
Raw almonds (1 cup)
Agave nectar (4 TB.)
Light coconut milk (1 cup)
Diced tomatoes (2 [14.5 oz.; 411g cans])
Tomato paste (¼ cup + 1 TB.)
Chickpeas (2 [15-oz.; 425g] cans)
Black beans (1 [15-oz.; 425g] can)
Purified water (10 qt.; 10l)
Loose-leaf black tea, decaffeinated (2 TB.)
Vanilla (2 tsp.)
Cumin (2 TB. + 2 tsp.)
Cinnamon (1 TB. + ½ tsp.)
Cayenne (½ tsp.)
Paprika (1 tsp.)
Curry powder (2 tsp.)
Cinnamon sticks (2)
Star anise (1)
Ground cardamom (¾ tsp.)
Ancho chile powder (1 TB. + 1½ tsp.)
Chile de árbol (3 TB.)
Chili powder (½ TB.)
Salt
Pepper

PREPARATION			DURING THE CLEANSE	
1 WEEK BEFORE	**3 DAYS BEFORE**	**1 DAY BEFORE**	**DAILY SOUPS**	**CLEANSE BOOSTERS**
★ Make **Vuelve a la Vida Broth** (single batch); freeze in 2-cup portions. RECIPE PAGE 182	★ Make **Curried Butternut Soup** (double batch); refrigerate in 2-cup portions. RECIPE PAGE 91	★ Make **Mango Soup with Lime** (double batch); refrigerate in 2-cup portions. RECIPE PAGE 27	**BREAKFAST** Mango Soup with Lime (2 cups)	★ Drink 2 cups of alkalized water between meals.
★ Make **Black Bean Poblano Soup** (single batch); freeze in 2-cup portions. RECIPE PAGE 102	★ Make **Spiced Chickpea Soup** (double batch); refrigerate in 2-cup portions. RECIPE PAGE 137	★ Make **Chai Spiced Almond Soup** (double batch); refrigerate in 1-cup portions. RECIPE PAGE 140	**SNACK** Vuelve a la Vida Broth (2 cups)	★ Perform 30 to 60 minutes of moderate exercise daily during cleanse, particularly HIIT routines or weight training.
★ Eliminate processed foods and sugar from your diet and focus on whole foods.	★ Eliminate poultry, meat, and dairy from your diet.	★ Transfer Vuelve a la Vida Broth and Black Bean Poblano Soup from freezer to refrigerator to thaw.	**LUNCH** Black Bean Poblano Soup (2 cups)	★ Receive a colonic treatment halfway through or at the end of your cleanse.
	★ Focus on vegetable-based meals supplemented with fish, grains, and legumes.	★ Eliminate all animal products from your diet.	**SNACK** Curried Butternut Soup (2 cups)	
		★ Eat vegetable-based meals with some legumes, grains, and nuts.	**DINNER** Spiced Chickpea Soup (2 cups)	
		★ Drink at least 8 cups of water.	**DESSERT** Chai Spiced Almond Soup (1 cup)	
			ALTERNATIVES Cantaloupe Jalapeño Soup (breakfast) RECIPE PAGE 61	
			Jalapeño Chicken Broth (snack) RECIPE PAGE 156	

KIWI KALE GAZPACHO

Slightly **tart and refreshing,** this soup features a variety of **vitamin-packed** fruits and leafy greens. **Sweet grapes** and **tangy kiwi** balance the earthier flavors of spinach and kale. Serve chilled.

 PREP & COOK
10 minutes

 QUANTITY
Makes 2 cups
Serving size 1 cup

 STORAGE
Refrigerated 5 days
Frozen 8 weeks

INGREDIENTS

1 cup kiwi, peeled and chopped

½ cup kale, chopped and stems removed

½ cup green grapes, halved

½ cup baby spinach

½ cup filtered water

2 tsp. agave nectar

METHOD

1 Place kiwi, kale, grapes, spinach, water, and agave nectar in blender. Purée for 30 seconds or until smooth.

2 If desired, transfer blending vessel to refrigerator to chill for 30 minutes. Blend briefly before serving.

NUTRITION PER SERVING

calories	114
total fat	1g
cholesterol	0mg
sodium	16mg
carbohydrate	27g
dietary fiber	4g
sugars	19g
protein	2g

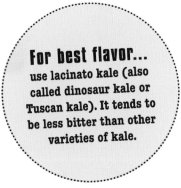

For best flavor... use lacinato kale (also called dinosaur kale or Tuscan kale). It tends to be less bitter than other varieties of kale.

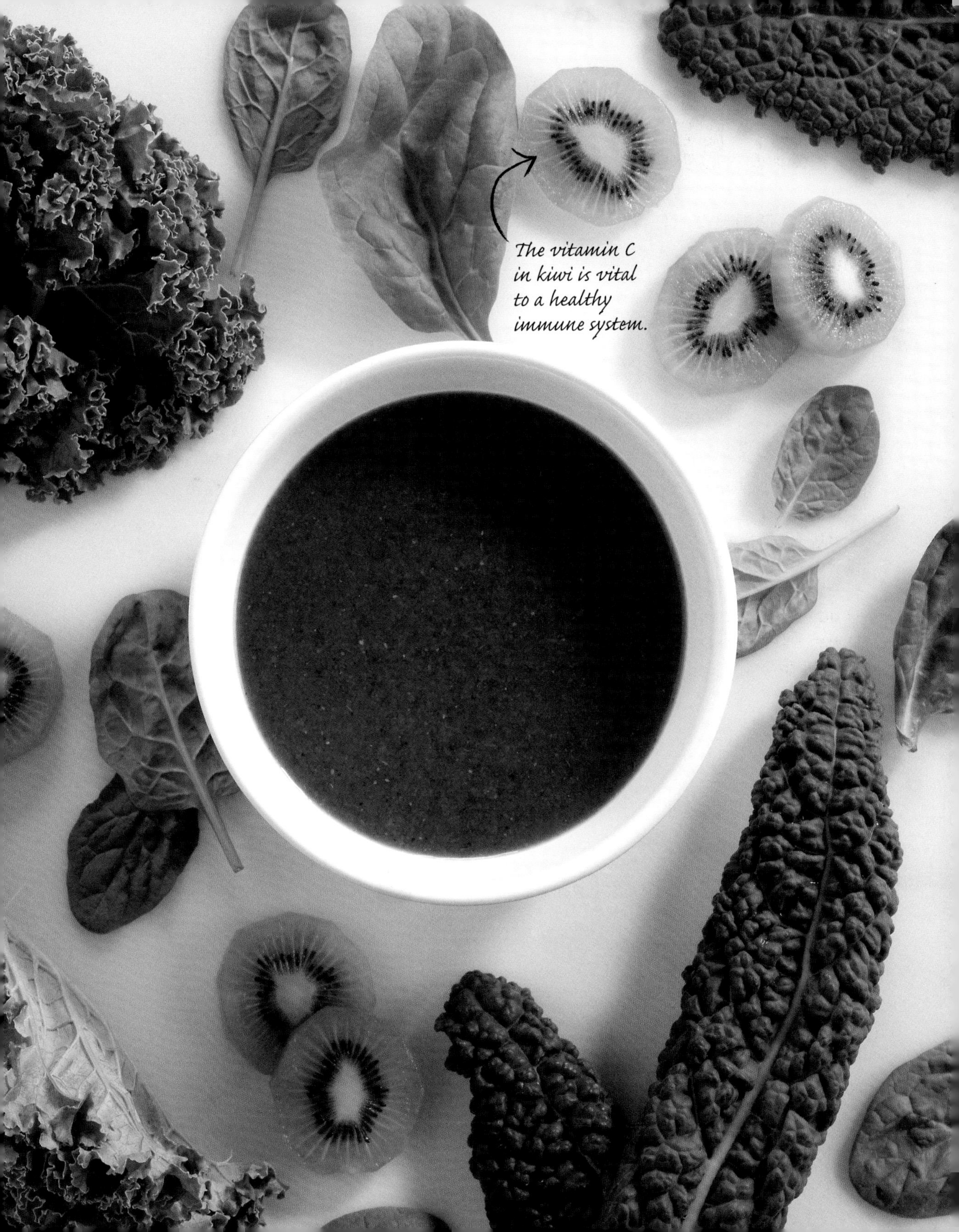

The vitamin C
in kiwi is vital
to a healthy
immune system.

CURRIED CARROT SOUP

Coconut milk and curry pair with **sweet carrots** and **spicy ginger** in this **savory, warming soup.** Rich in vitamins A and C, this soup is both nutritious and restorative. Serve hot.

 PREP & COOK
30 minutes

 QUANTITY
Makes 4 cups
Serving size 2 cups

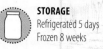 **STORAGE**
Refrigerated 5 days
Frozen 8 weeks

INGREDIENTS

¾ TB. coconut oil

¾ cup onion, diced

¾ tsp. garlic, minced

2 cups carrot, peeled and diced

4 cups purified water

1 tsp. curry powder

¼ cup light coconut milk

¼ tsp. fresh ginger, grated

⅛ tsp. salt

⅛ tsp. pepper

METHOD

1 In a medium pot, heat coconut oil over medium heat for 2 minutes.

2 Add onion and garlic and cook for 5 minutes or until garlic is fragrant and onions are translucent.

3 Add carrots and water to pot, increase heat, and bring to a boil. Reduce heat, cover, and simmer until carrots are tender, about 10 minutes.

4 Transfer contents of pot to blender and add curry powder, coconut milk, and grated ginger. Carefully blend for 30 seconds or until smooth. Add salt and pepper to taste.

NUTRITION PER SERVING

calories	166
total fat	9g
cholesterol	0mg
sodium	242mg
carbohydrate	22g
dietary fiber	7g
sugars	10g
protein	3g

Stir in...
1 TB. chia seeds just before serving for added protein and texture.

ZUCCHINI POBLANO SOUP

The **smokey, mildly spicy poblano** pepper shines in this recipe, while fiber-rich zucchini provides a silky base. **Lime and cumin** round out the **Latin flavor** of this **zesty, satisfying soup.** Serve hot.

PREP & COOK
25 minutes

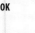

QUANTITY
Makes 6 cups
Serving size 2 cups

STORAGE
Refrigerated 5 days
Frozen 8 weeks

INGREDIENTS

1½ tsp. coconut oil

1 cup onion, diced

2 tsp. serrano pepper, minced

2 cups poblano pepper, diced and seeds removed

¼ cup corn kernels

4 cups zucchini, chopped

4½ cups purified water

½ cup cilantro, chopped and stems removed

Juice of 2 limes

½ tsp. cumin

⅛ tsp. salt

⅛ tsp. pepper

METHOD

1 In a medium pot, heat coconut oil over medium heat for 2 minutes. Add onion, serrano, and poblano. Cook until onion is translucent, about 5 minutes.

2 Add corn, zucchini, and water and bring to a boil. Reduce heat and simmer for 7 minutes or until vegetables are cooked through. Remove from heat.

3 Transfer contents of pot to blender and add cilantro, lime juice, and cumin. Purée for 30 seconds or until smooth, adding water to thin as needed. Season with salt and pepper.

NUTRITION PER SERVING

calories	167
total fat	3g
cholesterol	0mg
sodium	140mg
carbohydrate	33g
dietary fiber	8g
sugars	17g
protein	7g

BEET, ORANGE, & BASIL SOUP

This ruby-hued soup combines the **subtle earthiness** of beets with the **bright sweetness** of orange and **herbal notes** of fresh basil for a meal that is both **detoxifying and energizing.** Serve chilled.

 PREP & COOK
1 hour 15 minutes

 QUANTITY
Makes 4 cups
Serving size 2 cups

 STORAGE
Refrigerated 4 days
Frozen 8 weeks

INGREDIENTS

2 medium beets, ends removed

1 TB. olive oil

1½ cups freshly squeezed orange juice

1 tsp. red onion, chopped

½ cup fresh basil, minced

1 tsp. fresh ginger, grated

1 cup purified water

METHOD

1 Preheat oven to 450°F (230°C). Line a baking sheet with foil. Place beets on prepared baking sheet, drizzle with olive oil, and roast for 20 to 45 minutes or until cooked through and fork-tender.

2 Remove beets from oven, carefully peel, and cut into cubes. (You should have about 2 cups roasted beets.)

3 In a blender, combine roasted beets, orange juice, onion, basil, ginger, and water. Purée for 30 seconds.

4 Transfer blending vessel to refrigerator for 30 minutes or until chilled. Blend briefly to recombine ingredients and serve immediately.

NUTRITION PER SERVING

calories	183
total fat	7g
cholesterol	0mg
sodium	66mg
carbohydrate	29g
dietary fiber	3g
sugars	21g
protein	3g

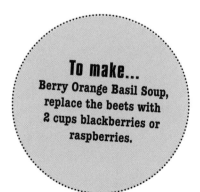
To make...
Berry Orange Basil Soup, replace the beets with 2 cups blackberries or raspberries.

Beets are high in folate, which is vital to healthy cell growth.

SPINACH & WHITE BEAN SOUP

Hearty and filling, this soup features a savory base of onion, carrot, and celery, with **white beans for body and protein.** Fresh basil, garlic, and lemon complement the **earthy greens.** Serve hot.

 PREP & COOK
35 minutes

 QUANTITY
Makes 6 cups
Serving size 2 cups

STORAGE
Refrigerated 5 days
Frozen 8 weeks

INGREDIENTS

¾ TB. olive oil
¾ cup onion, diced
¾ cup carrot, diced
¾ cup celery, diced
3 cloves garlic, minced
1 TB. tomato paste
5 cups purified water
2 (15-oz.; 425g) cans Great
   Northern beans, drained
   and rinsed
2 cups baby spinach
1 cup kale, roughly chopped
¼ tsp. red pepper flakes
3 TB. fresh basil, chopped
1 tsp. lemon juice
⅛ tsp. salt
⅛ tsp. pepper

METHOD

1 In a medium pot, heat olive oil over medium heat for 2 minutes or until shimmering.

2 Add onion, carrots, celery, and garlic and cook for 5 minutes or until garlic is fragrant and onions are translucent. Add tomato paste and cook for another 5 minutes.

3 Add water and beans, increase heat, and bring to a boil. Reduce heat and simmer for 10 minutes. Stir in spinach and kale and allow to wilt.

4 Carefully transfer contents of pot to blender. Add red pepper flakes, basil, and lemon juice. Purée for 30 seconds or until smooth. Season with salt and pepper.

Instead of water... use chicken bone broth for a richer flavor profile and added health benefits.

NUTRITION PER SERVING

calories	262	carbohydrate	48g
total fat	2g	dietary fiber	11g
cholesterol	0mg	sugars	5g
sodium	171mg	protein	15g

SPRING VEGETABLE SOUP

A **slow-simmered vegetable broth** forms the base of this delicate soup. **Shaved carrot** and **thinly sliced fennel** mingle with baby spinach and spring peas for the **perfect light afternoon meal.** Serve hot.

PREP & COOK
1 hour 35 minutes

QUANTITY
Makes 4 cups
Serving size 2 cups

STORAGE
Refrigerated 5 days
Frozen 8 weeks

INGREDIENTS

For Vegetable Broth:

2 tsp. olive oil

¾ cup onion, roughly chopped

¾ cup carrot, roughly chopped

¾ cup celery, roughly chopped

3 cloves garlic, peeled

8 cups purified water

1 cup parsley, stems and leaves, lightly packed

For Soup:

2 tsp. olive oil

¾ cup leek, rinsed and diced

1 tsp. garlic, minced (about 1 clove)

¼ cup carrot, peeled into long strips

1 cup baby spinach, tightly packed

¼ cup fennel, cut into ¼-inch (.5cm) slices

4 TB. frozen green peas

⅛ tsp. salt

⅛ tsp. pepper

METHOD

1 To make vegetable broth, in a medium stockpot, heat olive oil over medium heat for 2 minutes. Add onion, carrots, celery, and garlic and cook for 5 minutes or until onions are translucent. Add water and parsley. Cover, raise heat to high, and bring to a boil.

2 Reduce heat and simmer for 45 minutes to an hour. Strain vegetables from broth. (Vegetables can be discarded.)

3 To make soup, in a medium stockpot, heat olive oil over medium heat for 2 minutes. Add leek and garlic and cook until leek is soft, about 4 minutes.

4 Add vegetable broth, carrot, fennel, spinach, and frozen peas. Continue to cook over medium heat until vegetables are cooked through, about 5 minutes. Season with salt and pepper.

NUTRITION PER SERVING

calories	130	carbohydrate	24g
total fat	3g	dietary fiber	7g
cholesterol	0mg	sugars	9g
sodium	283mg	protein	5g

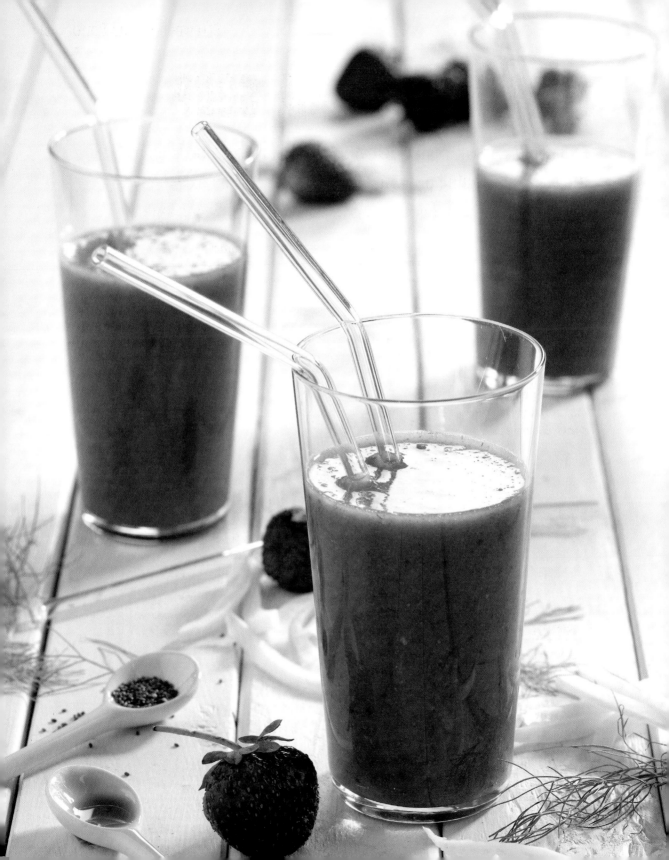

STRAWBERRY CHIA SOUP

Start your day with this **slightly sweet and refreshing** combination. Chia provides **filling protein,** strawberries contribute **key antioxidants,** and fennel lends **a savory balance.** Serve chilled.

 PREP & COOK
8 minutes

 QUANTITY
Makes 4 cups
Serving size 2 cups

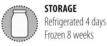 **STORAGE**
Refrigerated 4 days
Frozen 8 weeks

INGREDIENTS

2 cups fennel, diced

2 cups strawberries, hulled and halved

2 cups coconut water

1½ tsp. agave nectar

2 tsp. chia seeds

METHOD

1 In a blender, combine fennel, strawberries, coconut water, and agave nectar. Purée for 30 seconds or until smooth.

2 Stir in chia seeds and let sit for 10 minutes or until soup is slightly thickened.

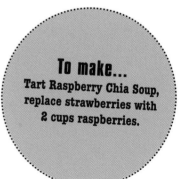

To make...
Tart Raspberry Chia Soup,
replace strawberries with
2 cups raspberries.

NUTRITION PER SERVING

calories	187
total fat	4g
cholesterol	0mg
sodium	301mg
carbohydrate	36g
dietary fiber	12g
sugars	21g
protein	5g

ENERGIZE
3-DAY CLEANSE

The soups in this cleanse are packed with ingredients that both boost energy and provide sustenance for long periods of time, making it the perfect cleanse for times you're feeling lethargic or depleted.

Follow for 3 days. After your cleanse, try incorporating these energy-boosting soups into your diet when you need an extra lift.

Shopping List

Fridge/Freezer
Carrots (11 medium)
Celery (10 stalks)
Kale, chopped (1 cup)
Baby spinach (4 cups)
Mushrooms (8 oz.; 227g)
Celeriac (2 bulbs)
Onion (10¼ cups)
Granny Smith apples (3)
Strawberries (4 cups)
Oranges (3)
Grapefruits (2)
Lemons (10)
Lemon juice (1 tsp.)
Garlic (17 cloves)
Chives (1 cup + 6 TB.)
Basil, chopped (3 TB.)
Fresh parsley (1½ cups)
Lavender, minced (2 tsp.)
Unsweetened almond milk (2 cups)
Greek yogurt, 2% plain (1 cup)

Pantry
Coconut water (⅔ cup)
Coconut oil (3 TB.)
Olive oil (1¼ cups)
Purified water (25 cups)
Tamari (4 TB.)
Vanilla extract (2 tsp.)
Honey (2 tsp.)
Flax seed, ground (4 TB.)
Chia seeds (2 TB.)
Goji berries, dried (6 TB.)
Freekeh (½ cup dry)
Tomato paste (1 TB.)
White beans (2 [15 oz.; 425g] cans)
Red pepper flakes (¼ tsp.)
Dried parsley (2 TB.)
Bay leaves (2)
Salt
Pepper

PREPARATION			DURING THE CLEANSE	
1 WEEK BEFORE	**3 DAYS BEFORE**	**1 DAY BEFORE**	**DAILY SOUPS**	**CLEANSE BOOSTERS**
★ Make **Tamari & Lemon Broth** (double batch); freeze in 2-cup portions. RECIPE PAGE 171	★ Make **Carrot Soup with Chives** (double batch); refrigerate in 2-cup portions. RECIPE PAGE 52	★ Make **Superfood Berry Soup** (double batch); refrigerate in 2-cup portions. RECIPE PAGE 31	**BREAKFAST** Superfood Berry Soup (2 cups)	★ Drink 2 cups of alkalized water between meals.
★ Make **Spinach & White Bean Soup** (single batch); freeze in 2-cup portions. RECIPE PAGE 42	★ Make **Apple & Celeriac Soup** (triple batch); refrigerate in 2-cup portions. RECIPE PAGE 109	★ Make **Citrus Soup with Lavender** (single batch); refrigerate in 1-cup portions. RECIPE PAGE 150	**SNACK** Tamari & Lemon Broth (2 cups)	★ Perform 20 to 30 minutes of light to moderate exercise daily.
★ Eliminate processed foods and sugar from your diet and focus on whole foods.	★ Eliminate poultry, meat, and dairy from your diet.	★ Transfer Tamari & Lemon Broth and Spinach & White Bean Soup from freezer to refrigerator to thaw.	**LUNCH** Carrot Soup with Chives (2 cups)	★ Receive a colonic treatment halfway through or at the end of your cleanse.
	★ Focus on vegetable-based meals supplemented with fish, grains, and legumes.	★ Eliminate all animal products from your diet.	**SNACK** Apple & Celeriac Soup (2 cups)	
		★ Eat vegetable-based meals with some legumes, grains, and nuts.	**DINNER** Spinach & White Bean Soup (2 cups)	
		★ Drink at least 8 cups of water.	**DESSERT** Citrus Soup with Lavender (1 cup)	
			ALTERNATIVES Apple & Amaranth Soup (breakfast) RECIPE PAGE 100	
			Banana Walnut Soup (snack) RECIPE PAGE 107	

GINGER GREENS SOUP

Coconut milk gives this **light and hydrating combination** a silky texture, which is accented by a **touch of ginger**. Romaine and spinach lend a **fresh, vegetal flavor** and deep, verdant color. Serve chilled.

 PREP & COOK
40 minutes

 QUANTITY
Makes 4 cups
Serving size 2 cups

 STORAGE
Refrigerated 4 days
Frozen 8 weeks

INGREDIENTS

¾ TB. olive oil
1 cup onion, diced
2 tsp. garlic, minced
    (about 2 cloves)
2 cups romaine, roughly
    chopped
2 cups baby spinach,
    tightly packed
¼ cup cilantro, tightly
    packed
2 cups purified water
1 tsp. fresh ginger, grated
⅛ cup light coconut milk
⅛ tsp. salt
⅛ tsp. pepper

METHOD

1 In a medium pan, heat olive oil over medium for 2 minutes. Add onion and garlic, and cook until onion is translucent, about 5 minutes.

2 Transfer onion and garlic to blender. Add romaine, spinach, cilantro, water, and ginger. Purée for 30 seconds. Add coconut milk and season with salt and pepper. Blend until smooth.

3 Transfer blending vessel to refrigerator for 30 minutes or until chilled. Blend briefly before serving to recombine ingredients.

superfood spinach is full of nutrients, including fiber, calcium, and potassium.

To make...
Savory Sesame Greens Soup, add 1 TB. tamari and ½ tsp. sesame oil to the blender.

NUTRITION PER SERVING

calories	67
total fat	2g
cholesterol	0mg
sodium	195mg
carbohydrate	12g
dietary fiber	3g
sugars	5g
protein	3g

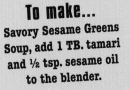

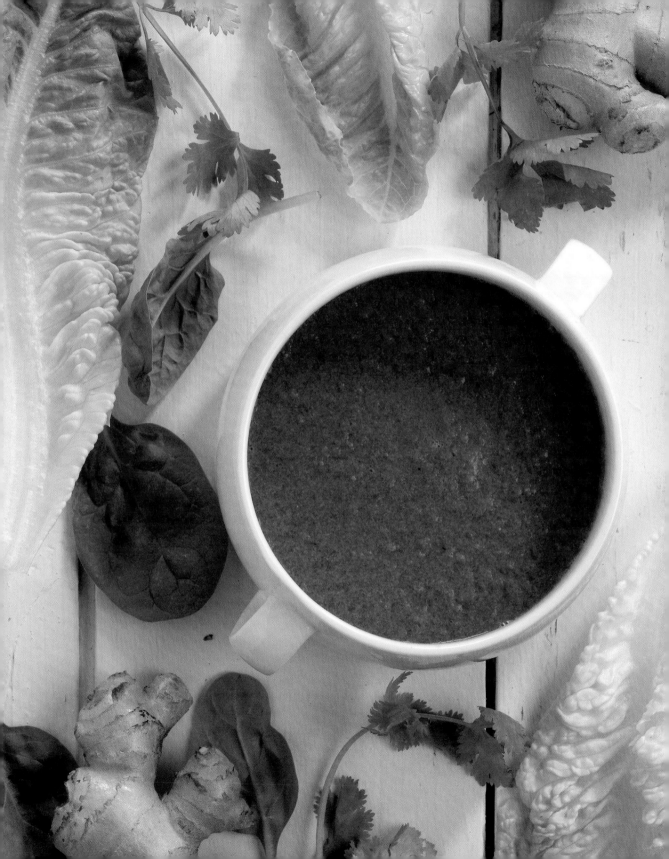

Asparagus is high in vitamin K, which helps build healthy bones and protects against heart disease.

ASPARAGUS SOUP WITH MINT

This **light, savory soup** captures the **taste of spring**. The fresh flavor of asparagus is highlighted by **cool mint** and **zesty lemon**. Smooth and refreshing, this soup is a **perfect afternoon boost**. Serve chilled.

PREP & COOK
20 minutes

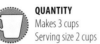
QUANTITY
Makes 3 cups
Serving size 2 cups

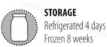
STORAGE
Refrigerated 4 days
Frozen 8 weeks

INGREDIENTS

¾ TB. olive oil

1 tsp. garlic, minced

1 cup onion, diced

2 cups asparagus, trimmed and chopped

½ cup baby spinach, tightly packed

¼ tsp. lemon zest

½ tsp. mint, chopped

1½ cups cold purified water

¼ tsp. salt

METHOD

1 In a small pan, heat olive oil over medium heat for 2 minutes. Add onion and garlic, and cook until onion is translucent, about 5 minutes. Remove from heat.

2 Prepare an ice bath by filling a medium bowl with water and ice cubes.

3 Fill a saucepan halfway with water and bring to a boil over high heat. Blanch asparagus by submerging in boiling water for 30 seconds. Remove from heat, drain, and quickly plunge asparagus in ice bath. Let sit for 5 minutes.

4 Drain asparagus and add to blender along with onion, garlic, spinach, lemon zest, mint, water, and salt. Purée until asparagus is well processed and smooth.

NUTRITION PER SERVING

calories	97
total fat	2g
cholesterol	0mg
sodium	405mg
carbohydrate	18g
dietary fiber	6g
sugars	8g
protein	6g

For a heartier soup...
use chicken bone broth instead of water, and top with ¼ cup sautéed mushrooms.

CARROT SOUP WITH CHIVES

The **ancient supergrain** freekeh lends a **nutty flavor** to this hearty soup, as well as a **boost of protein and fiber**. Top with a **swirl of chive oil** for an added savory note. Serve hot.

PREP & COOK
35 minutes

QUANTITY
Makes 3 cups
Serving size 2 cups

STORAGE
Refrigerated 6 days
Frozen 8 weeks

INGREDIENTS

1 tsp. + ½ cup olive oil

3 cups yellow onion, chopped

1 TB. garlic, minced (about 3 cloves)

1 cup carrot, peeled and chopped

1 cup filtered water

1 cup freekeh, cooked

2 cups chives, chopped

½ tsp. salt

½ tsp. pepper

METHOD

1 In a medium saucepan, heat 1 tsp. olive oil over medium heat. Add onion and garlic and cook for 5 minutes or until garlic is fragrant and onions are translucent.

2 Add carrots and water to saucepan and bring to a boil. Reduce heat to medium-low and simmer for 15 minutes or until carrots are cooked through.

3 Transfer contents of saucepan to blender and add water and cooked freekeh. Purée for 45 seconds or until smooth.

4 To make chive oil, combine chives, remaining ½ cup olive oil, salt, and pepper in a clean blender. Purée until oil is smooth and chives are fully incorporated.

5 Swirl 1 to 2 tsp. chive oil into soup before serving. (Leftover chive oil can be frozen for later use.)

NUTRITION PER SERVING

calories	346
total fat	8g
cholesterol	0mg
sodium	852mg
carbohydrate	64g
dietary fiber	14g
sugars	18g
protein	10g

Carrots are high in vitamin A, which helps promote strong bones and immune system health.

STRAWBERRY RHUBARB SOUP

Sweet and creamy, this blend is **reminiscent of a strawberry milkshake.** With fresh strawberries, tart rhubarb, and rich macadamia nuts, it **tastes indulgent** but delivers on nutrition. Serve chilled.

PREP & COOK
1 hour 10 minutes

QUANTITY
Makes 4 cups
Serving size 1 cup

STORAGE
Refrigerated 4 days
Frozen 8 weeks

INGREDIENTS

¾ cup unsalted macadamia nuts

⅔ cup rhubarb, diced

1 cup strawberries, hulled and halved

2⅔ cups purified water

2 TB. agave nectar

⅛ tsp. pepper

METHOD

1 Place macadamia nuts in a medium bowl and add hot water to cover. Let soak for 30 minutes to 24 hours before draining (discard soaking water).

2 In a small saucepan, bring ⅔ cup water to a boil over high heat. Add rhubarb and boil for 5 minutes or until tender. Drain and discard boiling water.

3 In a blender, combine macadamia nuts, rhubarb, strawberries, remaining 2 cups water, and agave nectar. Blend until nuts are broken down and mixture is smooth, about 45 seconds.

4 Transfer blending vessel to refrigerator for 30 minutes or until chilled. Blend briefly before serving.

NUTRITION PER SERVING

calories	227
total fat	19g
cholesterol	0mg
sodium	2mg
carbohydrate	15g
dietary fiber	3g
sugars	11g
protein	2g

To make...
Nut-Free Strawberry Rhubarb Soup, omit the macadamia nuts and add ¾ cup coconut milk yogurt to blender.

Agave nectar is less likely to cause blood sugar spikes than other sweeteners.

Macadamia nuts give this soup richness and body, as well as a nutritional boost of manganese.

3
SUMMER SOUPING

Summer souping features a weight loss cleanse and a cleanse for hydration. The vibrant flavors of summer ingredients are featured in a variety of chilled and raw soups, which will cool and hydrate your body while satisfying cravings.

BEET SOUP WITH FENNEL

The **robust flavor of beets** is complemented by fennel, lime, and ginger in this cleansing blend. **Earthy and slightly sweet,** this soup is **rich in folate and manganese** as well as vitamin C. Serve chilled.

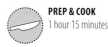
PREP & COOK
1 hour 15 minutes

QUANTITY
Makes 4 cups
Serving size 2 cups

STORAGE
Refrigerated 5 days
Frozen 8 weeks

INGREDIENTS

1 medium beet, ends removed

1 cup fennel, bulb and fronds, diced

Juice of 3 limes

2 tsp. mint, minced

2 tsp. fresh ginger, grated

2½ cups coconut water

METHOD

1 Preheat oven to 450°F (230°C). Line a baking sheet with foil. Place beet on prepared baking sheet, drizzle with olive oil, and roast for 30 to 40 minutes or until cooked through and tender.

2 Remove beet from oven, carefully peel, and cut into cubes. (You should have about 1 cup roasted beets.)

3 In a blender, combine roasted beets, fennel, lime juice, mint, ginger, and coconut water. Purée for 30 seconds.

4 Transfer blending vessel to refrigerator for 30 minutes or until chilled. Blend briefly to recombine before serving.

NUTRITION PER SERVING

calories	119
total fat	1g
cholesterol	0mg
sodium	315mg
carbohydrate	27g
dietary fiber	7g
sugars	15g
protein	4g

To make...
Citrus Fennel Ginger Soup, replace the roasted beets with 1½ cups orange or grapefruit segments.

3

SUMMER SOUPING

Summer souping features a weight loss cleanse and a cleanse for hydration. The vibrant flavors of summer ingredients are featured in a variety of chilled and raw soups, which will cool and hydrate your body while satisfying cravings.

For a refreshing tonic, try stirring a few tablespoons of soup into a glass of alkalized water.

Jalapeños are high in vitamin C, which helps build collagen, a critical connective tissue.

CANTALOUPE JALAPEÑO SOUP

In this soup, **juicy cantaloupe** pairs with **spicy jalapeño** and fresh basil to make a **refreshing combination** that reduces inflammation, **aids in digestion,** and **rehydrates the body.** Serve chilled.

PREP & COOK
45 minutes

QUANTITY
Makes 6 cups
Serving size 2 cups

STORAGE
Refrigerated 4 days
Frozen 8 weeks

INGREDIENTS

6 cups cantaloupe, cubed

1 tsp. jalapeño pepper, seeds removed and minced

½ cup fresh basil, chopped

2 cups purified water

2 TB. lime juice

METHOD

1 In a blender, combine cantaloupe, jalapeño, basil, water, and lime juice. Purée for 30 seconds or until smooth.

2 Transfer blending vessel to refrigerator for 30 minutes to chill. Before serving, season with salt and pepper and briefly blend to recombine ingredients, if needed.

Heat levels...
of jalapeños vary from pepper to pepper; add more or less based on the heat level of your peppers.

NUTRITION PER SERVING

calories	111
total fat	0g
cholesterol	0mg
sodium	55mg
carbohydrate	27g
dietary fiber	3g
sugars	25g
protein	3g

Cayenne stimulates circulation and boosts metabolic function.

RED PEPPER ROMESCO SOUP

In this summery soup, **sweet roasted peppers** are balanced by **tangy red wine vinegar** and spicy cayenne, while **protein-rich almonds** provide a **smooth, creamy texture.** Serve hot.

PREP & COOK
17 minutes

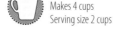

QUANTITY
Makes 4 cups
Serving size 2 cups

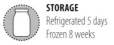

STORAGE
Refrigerated 5 days
Frozen 8 weeks

INGREDIENTS

2 TB. + 1 tsp. olive oil

1½ cups onion, diced

1 TB. garlic, minced
(about 3 cloves)

1 cup canned diced
tomatoes

3 cups roasted red peppers,
rinsed and drained

½ cup blanched almonds

⅔ tsp. cayenne

2 tsp. red wine vinegar

1 cup purified water

⅛ tsp. salt

⅛ tsp. pepper

METHOD

1 In a medium pan, heat 2 TB. olive oil over medium heat for 2 minutes. Add onion and garlic, and cook for 5 minutes or until onion is translucent.

2 Transfer onion and garlic to blender. Add diced tomatoes, roasted red peppers, almonds, cayenne, red wine vinegar, water, and remaining 1 tsp. olive oil.

3 Blend until ingredients are smooth and well combined. Season with salt and pepper and heat before serving.

NUTRITION PER SERVING

calories	308
total fat	14g
cholesterol	0mg
sodium	240mg
carbohydrate	40g
dietary fiber	12g
sugars	21g
protein	11g

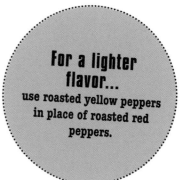

For a lighter
flavor...
use roasted yellow peppers
in place of roasted red
peppers.

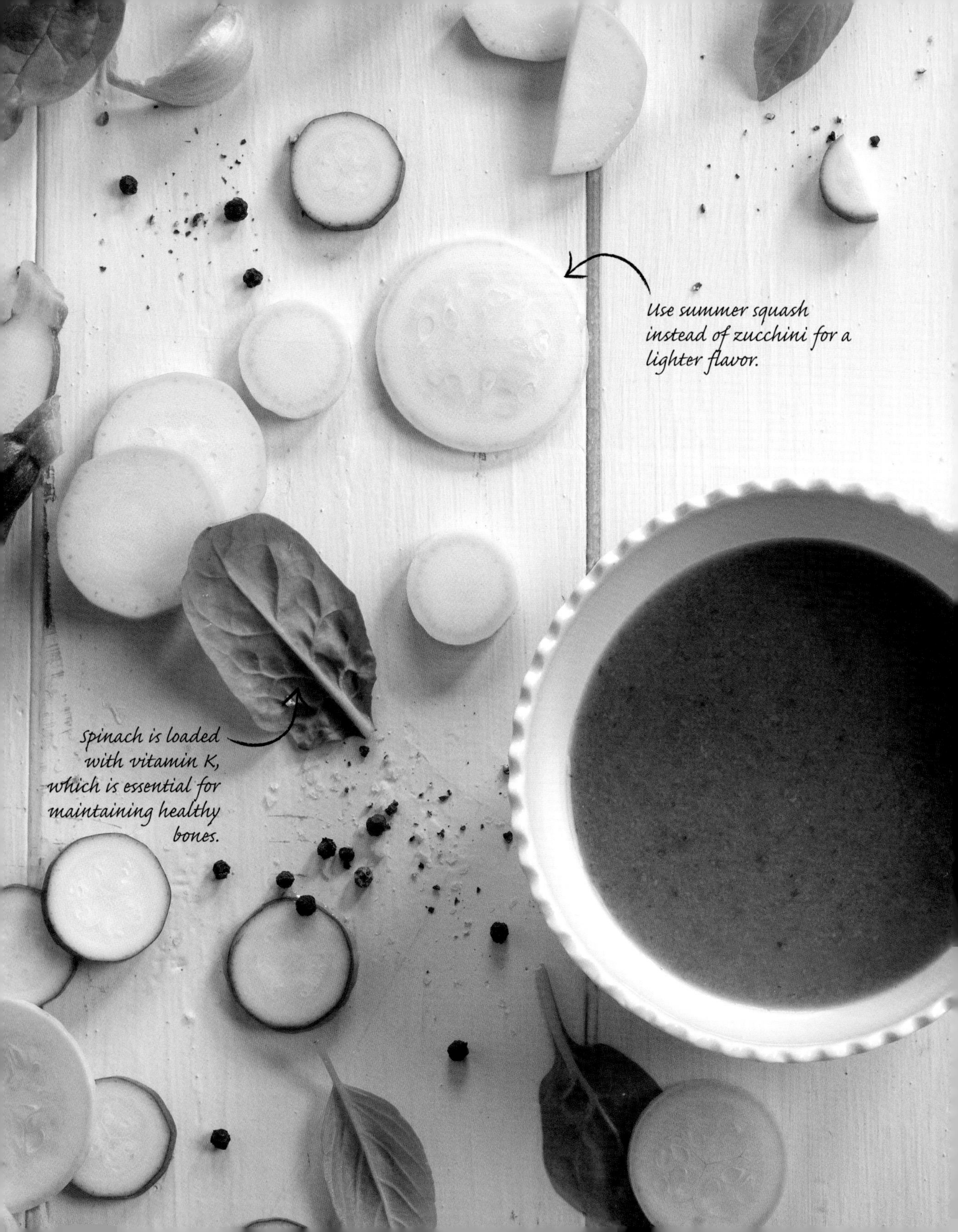

Use summer squash
instead of zucchini for a
lighter flavor.

Spinach is loaded
with vitamin K,
which is essential for
maintaining healthy
bones.

ZUCCHINI SOUP WITH BASIL

Puréed zucchini gives this soup a **delicate flavor** and **silky texture,** which is **enhanced by savory onion** and floral basil. Light but satisfying, it is a **perfect summer lunch.** Serve hot.

 PREP & COOK
25 minutes

 QUANTITY
Makes 6 cups
Serving size 2 cups

 STORAGE
Refrigerated 5 days
Frozen 8 weeks

INGREDIENTS

¾ TB. olive oil

1 cup onion, diced

2 tsp. garlic, minced
(about 2 cloves)

4 cups zucchini or summer
squash, roughly chopped

6 cups purified water

1 cup baby spinach, tightly
packed

4 TB. fresh basil, chopped

⅛ tsp. salt

⅛ tsp. pepper

METHOD

1 In a medium stockpot, heat olive oil over medium heat for 2 minutes. Add onion and garlic, and cook until onion is translucent, about 5 minutes.

2 Add zucchini and water, and bring to a boil. Reduce heat and simmer for 10 minutes or until zucchini is cooked through. Remove 2 cups cooking water and set aside.

3 Carefully transfer contents of pot to blender. Add spinach and basil, and purée until well combined. Add reserved cooking water as needed to reach deisred consistency. Season with salt and pepper.

NUTRITION PER SERVING

calories	95
total fat	2g
cholesterol	0mg
sodium	133mg
carbohydrate	17g
dietary fiber	4g
sugars	10g
protein	5g

WEIGHT LOSS
5-DAY CLEANSE

While exercise is important when it comes to weight loss, nutrition is even more crucial. Just by making smart changes to your diet, you can impact your weight. Consistency is the key to lasting weight loss, but this cleanse is a great way to get started.

Follow for 5 days to kick-start your weight loss. Afterward, incorporate a 3-day cleanse on a weekly basis or incorporate soups individually into your daily diet for continued weight loss.

Shopping List

Fridge/Freezer
Baby spinach (3 cups)
Carrots (12 medium)
Onions (9 medium)
Leeks (3)
Celery (7 stalks)
Green onion (1 bunch)
Red bell pepper (2)
Poblano pepper (2)
Jalapeño pepper (1)
Sweet corn (8 ears)
Sweet potato (1)
Butternut squash (1 small)
Parsnip (3 medium)
Fennel (1 bulb)
Cantaloupes (2 large)
Limes (8)
Parsley (1 bunch)
Basil (1 cup, chopped)
Garlic (38 cloves)
Fresh ginger (2 large pieces)
Lemongrass (2 cups, chopped)
Cilantro (1 bunch)
Fresh thyme (1 tsp., minced)
Frozen peas (¾ cup)

Pantry
Olive oil (¾ cup)
Toasted sesame oil (2 tsp.)
Purified water (16 qt.; 16l)
Coconut oil (3 TB.)
Tamari (6 TB.)
Raw almonds (2 cups)
Cacao nibs (6 TB.)
Agave nectar (2 TB.)
Unsweetened coconut flakes (2 TB.)
Hemp seeds (8 TB.)
Cumin (1 tsp.)
Salt
Pepper

PREPARATION

DURING THE CLEANSE

1 WEEK BEFORE

3 DAYS BEFORE

1 DAY BEFORE

DAILY SOUPS

CLEANSE BOOSTERS

★ Make **Sesame Vegetable Broth;** freeze in 2-cup portions. RECIPE PAGE 158

★ Make **Winter Root Vegetable Soup;** freeze in 2-cup portions. RECIPE PAGE 131

★ Remove processed foods and sugar from your diet and focus on whole foods.

★ Make **Sweet Corn & Pepper Soup;** refrigerate in 2-cup portions. RECIPE PAGE 76

★ Make **Spring Vegetable Soup;** refrigerate in 2-cup portions. RECIPE PAGE 43

★ Eliminate poultry, meat, and dairy from your diet.

★ Focus on vegetable-based meals supplemented with fish, grains, and legumes.

★ Make **Cantaloupe Jalapeño Soup;** refrigerate in 2-cup portions. RECIPE PAGE 61

★ Make **Almond Cacao Soup;** refrigerate in 1-cup portions. RECIPE PAGE 95

★ Transfer Sesame Vegetable Broth and Winter Root Vegetable Soup from freezer to refrigerator to thaw.

★ Eliminate all animal products from your diet.

★ Eat vegetable-based meals with some legumes, grains, and nuts.

★ Drink at least 8 cups of water.

BREAKFAST
Cantaloupe Jalapeño Soup (2 cups)

SNACK
Sesame Vegetable Broth (2 cups)

LUNCH
Winter Root Vegetable Soup (2 cups)

SNACK
Sweet Corn & Pepper Soup (2 cups)

DINNER
Spring Vegetable Soup (2 cups)

DESSERT
Almond Cacao Soup (1 cup)

ALTERNATIVES
Watermelon Aloe Mint Soup (breakfast)
RECIPE PAGE 80

Spinach & White Bean Soup (snack)
RECIPE PAGE 42

★ Drink 2 cups of alkalized water between meals.

★ Perform 45 to 60 minutes of moderate exercise daily during cleanse, focusing on cardio workouts.

★ Receive a colonic treatment halfway through or at the end of your cleanse.

Chives contain potassium, which helps promote healthy kidney function.

SWEET CORN & CHIVE SOUP

This **lightly sweet purée** showcases **fresh summer corn,** which is an excellent source of **dietary fiber** and aids in digestion. Cool and refreshing, it is a **perfect light lunch** or snack. Serve chilled.

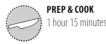 **PREP & COOK**
1 hour 15 minutes

 QUANTITY
Makes 6 cups
Serving size 2 cups

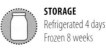 **STORAGE**
Refrigerated 4 days
Frozen 8 weeks

INGREDIENTS

2 TB. coconut oil

2 cups onion, chopped

2 tsp. garlic, minced
(about 2 cloves)

6 ears fresh sweet corn

6 cups purified water

1 tsp. salt

½ tsp. pepper

4 TB. chives, chopped

METHOD

1 In medium stockpot, heat coconut oil over medium heat. Add onion and garlic, and cook until onions are translucent, about 5 minutes.

2 Cut corn kernels from cobs. (You should have about 4 cups of corn.) Set aside 4 corn cobs.

3 Add water, corn kernels, and 4 corn cobs to pot, and bring to a boil. Reduce heat, cover, and simmer for 30 minutes.

4 Remove corn cobs and discard. Remove 1 cup cooking water and set aside. Transfer contents of pot to blender. Purée for 30 seconds or until smooth, adding reserved cooking water to thin if needed. Season with salt and pepper.

5 Transfer blending vessel to refrigerator for 30 minutes or until chilled. Stir in chopped chives just before serving.

NUTRITION PER SERVING

calories	293
total fat	12g
cholesterol	0mg
sodium	799mg
carbohydrate	47g
dietary fiber	5g
sugars	17g
protein	8g

To make...
Smokey Tomato & Corn Soup, add 2 cups fire-roasted diced tomatoes, 2 roasted red peppers, and 1 tsp. chipotle powder to blender.

PEACH SOUP WITH BASIL

With **ripe peaches** and coconut water, this **slightly sweet, herbal** combination **tastes like summer.** Lemon juice adds a tart note. For a sweeter flavor, add **a splash of agave nectar.** Serve chilled.

 PREP & COOK
10 minutes

 QUANTITY
Makes 6 cups
Serving size 2 cups

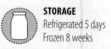 **STORAGE**
Refrigerated 5 days
Frozen 8 weeks

INGREDIENTS

5 large peaches, diced
  (about 4 cups)

½ cup fresh basil, julienned

3 cups coconut water

1 TB. lemon juice

METHOD

1 In a blender, combine peaches, basil, coconut water, and lemon juice. Purée for 30 seconds or until smooth.

2 If desired, transfer blending vessel to refrigerator for 30 minutes to chill. Blend briefly to recombine ingredients before serving.

To make...
Creamy Peach Soup with Mint, omit lemon juice, replace basil with fresh mint, and add 2 cups Greek yogurt.

NUTRITION PER SERVING

calories	149
total fat	1g
cholesterol	0mg
sodium	65mg
carbohydrate	36g
dietary fiber	4g
sugars	31g
protein	3g

PAPAYA & SPINACH SOUP

This **sweet combination** of **creamy papaya** and **fresh spinach** gets a nutrient boost from **spirulina,** an algae rich in protein, vitamins, and antioxidants. Lime and cilantro add a **zesty, herbal** note. Serve chilled.

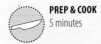 **PREP & COOK**
5 minutes

 QUANTITY
Makes 4 cups
Serving size 2 cups

 STORAGE
Refrigerated 5 days
Freezing not recommended

INGREDIENTS

3 cups papaya, cubed

2 cups baby spinach, lightly packed

¼ cup cilantro, chopped and stems removed

2 TB. lime juice

1½ cups coconut water

1½ tsp. spirulina powder

METHOD

1 In a blender, combine papaya, spinach, cilantro, lime juice, and coconut water. Purée for 30 seconds or until smooth.

2 Add spirulina powder to blender and blend until combined. If desired, transfer blending vessel to refrigerator to chill for 30 minutes before serving.

NUTRITION PER SERVING	
calories	158
total fat	1g
cholesterol	0mg
sodium	71mg
carbohydrate	36g
dietary fiber	4g
sugars	26g
protein	3g

HERBED CUCUMBER SOUP

With its **light, clean flavor** profile, this soup will keep you **cool and hydrated.** Fresh mint and dill add **herbal notes,** while lemon juice provides a **bright and balanced** tartness. Serve chilled.

 PREP & COOK
10 minutes

 QUANTITY
Makes 6 cups
Serving size 2 cups

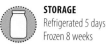 **STORAGE**
Refrigerated 5 days
Frozen 8 weeks

INGREDIENTS

5 cups English cucumber, peeled and chopped

3 cups purified water

⅔ cup green onion, chopped

¼ cup fresh dill, chopped

2 TB. fresh mint, chopped

Juice of 2 lemons

⅛ tsp. salt

⅛ tsp. pepper

METHOD

1 In a blender, combine cucumber, water, green onion, dill, mint, and lemon juice. Purée for 30 seconds.

2 If desired, transfer blending vessel to refrigerator for 30 minutes to chill. Before serving, add salt and pepper, and blend briefly to recombine ingredients, if needed.

NUTRITION PER SERVING

calories	47
total fat	1g
cholesterol	0mg
sodium	263mg
carbohydrate	10g
dietary fiber	3g
sugars	5g
protein	2g

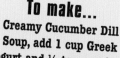

To make...
Creamy Cucumber Dill Soup, add 1 cup Greek yogurt and ½ tsp. cumin to blender, and replace lemon juice with lime juice.

For the smoothest texture, use seedless cucumbers, or remove the seeds before puréeing.

Mint is a digestive aid as well as a natural stimulant.

PEACHES & GREENS SOUP

Sweet peaches and tangy, tropical pineapple are enhanced by mint and ginger in this **refreshing, green blend**. Packed with **vitamins A and C** as well as fiber, this soup is **sure to satisfy**. Serve chilled.

 PREP & COOK
15 minutes

QUANTITY
Makes 5 cups
Serving size 2 cups

STORAGE
Refrigerated 4 days
Freezing not recommended

INGREDIENTS

2 cups cucumber, peeled and chopped

2 cups baby spinach, tightly packed

1½ cups peach, peeled and chopped

1½ cups pineapple, chopped

1 TB. fresh mint, minced

1 tsp. fresh ginger, grated

2 cups coconut water

METHOD

1 Place cucumber, spinach, peach, pineapple, mint, ginger, and coconut water in blender. Purée for 30 seconds or until smooth.

2 If desired, transfer blending vessel to refrigerator for 30 minutes to chill. Blend briefly before serving.

NUTRITION PER SERVING

calories	177
total fat	1g
cholesterol	0mg
sodium	281mg
carbohydrate	41g
dietary fiber	8g
sugars	30g
protein	5g

If peaches...
are not yet in season, use 1½ cups cubed mango instead.

ARTICHOKE BASIL SOUP

Artichokes give this soup a **luxurious, creamy texture** as well as a healthy dose of **antioxidants** and fiber. **Fragrant basil** and **zested lemon** add a crispness to this nutritional powerhouse. Serve hot.

PREP & COOK
35 minutes

QUANTITY
Makes 4 cups
Serving size 2 cups

STORAGE
Refrigerated 4 days
Frozen 8 weeks

INGREDIENTS

1 TB. coconut oil

⅓ cup onion, diced

⅓ cup carrot, diced

⅓ cup celery, diced

1 TB. garlic, minced (about 3 cloves)

1 (14-oz.; 400g) can artichoke hearts, rinsed and drained

3 cups purified water

2 cups baby spinach

½ cup fresh basil, chopped

1 TB. lemon zest

⅛ tsp. salt

⅛ tsp. pepper

METHOD

1 In a medium stockpot, heat coconut oil over medium heat for 2 minutes.

2 Add onion, carrots, celery, and garlic, and cook for 5 minutes or until garlic is fragrant and onions are translucent.

3 Add artichokes and water to pot, increase heat, and bring to a boil. Reduce heat and simmer for 10 minutes. Remove and reserve 1 cup cooking water. Stir in spinach.

4 Transfer soup to blender and add basil and lemon zest. Carefully blend until smooth, adding reserved cooking water to thin as needed. Season with salt and pepper.

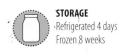

NUTRITION PER SERVING

calories	192	carbohydrate	30g
total fat	7g	dietary fiber	8g
cholestoral	0mg	sugars	1g
sodium	386mg	protein	9g

SWEET CORN & PEPPER SOUP

This **smokey, savory combination** of fresh sweet corn, red bell pepper, and poblano pepper is **reminiscent of corn chowder.** Simmering the corn cobs helps to flavor and thicken the soup. Serve hot.

 PREP & COOK
40 minutes

 QUANTITY
Makes 6 cups
Serving size 2 cups

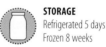 **STORAGE**
Refrigerated 5 days
Frozen 8 weeks

INGREDIENTS

1½ TB. olive oil

1 cup onion, diced

⅔ cup red bell pepper, diced

⅔ cup poblano pepper, diced

2 TB. garlic, minced (about 6 cloves)

4 ears fresh sweet corn

3½ cups purified water

½ tsp. cumin

3 TB. cilantro, chopped and stems removed

⅛ tsp. salt

⅛ tsp. pepper

METHOD

1 In a medium pot, heat olive oil over medium heat for 2 minutes. Add onion, red bell pepper, poblano pepper, and garlic. Cook until onion is translucent, about 5 minutes.

2 Cut corn kernels from cobs. (You should have about 3 cups of corn.) After removing kernels, set aside 2 corn cobs.

3 Add water, corn kernels, and 2 corn cobs to pot, and bring to a boil. Reduce heat, cover, and simmer for 15 minutes or until vegetables are cooked through and broth has thickened from the "milk" of the cobs. Remove from heat.

4 Remove corn cobs and transfer contents of pot to blender. Add cumin and cilantro and purée for 30 seconds or until smooth. Add salt and pepper and blend briefly before serving.

NUTRITION PER SERVING

calories	271
total fat	9g
cholesterol	0mg
sodium	152mg
carbohydrate	48g
dietary fiber	8g
sugars	14g
protein	8g

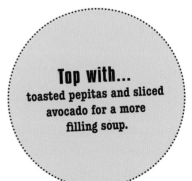

Top with...
toasted pepitas and sliced avocado for a more filling soup.

Red pepper contains vitamin E, which contributes to heart health.

HYDRATE
2-DAY CLEANSE

Staying hydrated is critical to keeping your body functioning at its best. While proper water intake is important, diet and lifestyle choices can also significantly impact the hydration levels of the body. If you've allowed yourself to become dehydrated, this regimen of soups will restore your body's balance.

Follow for 2 days. Get plenty of rest and avoid diuretics during the cleanse.

Shopping List

Fridge/Freezer

Celery (6 stalks)
Carrots (2 medium)
Garlic (8 cloves)
Onions (4)
Cucumbers (4)
Yellow bell pepper (1)
Kale (⅔ cup, chopped)
Avocado (1)
Cauliflower (1 small head)
Sunchokes (6)
Green onion (1 bunch)
Spinach (2 cups)
Lemons (7)
Pears (4)
Apples (2)
Peaches (2)
Pineapple (1½ cup, chopped)
Parsley (1 bunch)
Fresh basil (1 cup, chopped)
Fresh dill (¼ cup, chopped)
Mint (3 TB., minced)
Ginger (1 tsp., grated)

Pantry

Olive oil (3 TB.)
Palm sugar (1 TB.)
Coconut water (2 cups)
Purified water (5 qt.; 5l)
Bay leaf (1)
Cinnamon sticks (2)
Nutmeg (1 whole)
Cayenne (¼ tsp.)
Salt
Pepper

PREPARATION			DURING THE CLEANSE	
1 WEEK BEFORE	**3 DAYS BEFORE**	**1 DAY BEFORE**	**DAILY SOUPS**	**CLEANSE BOOSTERS**
★ Make **Vegetable Broth with Basil** (single batch); freeze in 2-cup portions. RECIPE PAGE 179	★ Make **Kale & Bell Pepper Soup** (single batch); refrigerate in 2-cup portions. RECIPE PAGE 33	★ Make **Herbed Cucumber Soup** (single batch); refrigerate in 2-cup portions. RECIPE PAGE 72	**BREAKFAST** Peaches & Greens Soup (2 cups)	★ Drink 2 cups of alkalized water between meals.
			SNACK Vegetable Broth with Basil (2 cups)	★ Sit in steam room for 15 to 20 minutes per day during your cleanse.
★ Make **Pear Soup with Cinnamon** (single batch); freeze in 1-cup portions. RECIPE PAGE 119	★ Make **Roasted Sunchoke Soup** (single batch); refrigerate in 2-cup portions. RECIPE PAGE 136	★ Make **Peaches & Greens Soup** (single batch); refrigerate in 2-cup portions. RECIPE PAGE 74	**LUNCH** Roasted Sunchoke Soup (2 cups)	
			SNACK Herbed Cucumber Soup (2 cups)	★ Get 7 to 8 hours of restful sleep nightly.
★ Eliminate processed foods and sugar from your diet and focus on whole foods.	★ Eliminate poultry, meat, and dairy from your diet.	★ Transfer Vegetable Broth with Basil and Pear Soup with Cinnamon from freezer to refrigerator to thaw.	**DINNER** Kale & Bell Pepper Soup (2 cups)	
			DESSERT Pear Soup with Cinnamon (1 cup)	
	★ Focus on vegetable-based meals supplemented with fish, grains, and legumes.	★ Eliminate all animal products from your diet.	**ALTERNATIVES** Avocado & Arugula Soup (dinner) RECIPE PAGE 29	
			Almond Cacao Soup (dessert) RECIPE PAGE 95	
		★ Eat vegetable-based meals with some legumes, grains, and nuts.		
		★ Drink at least 8 cups of water.		

WATERMELON ALOE MINT SOUP

The **light, fruity flavor of watermelon** meets **cooling aloe** in this wonderfully **refreshing and hydrating** soup. This blend **promotes healthy digestion** and reduces chronic inflammation. Serve chilled.

 PREP & COOK
10 minutes

 QUANTITY
Makes 4 cups
Serving size 2 cups

 STORAGE
Refrigerated 5 days
Freezing not recommended

INGREDIENTS

3 cups watermelon, cubed

Juice of 4 small lemons

2 TB. mint, chopped

1 cup pure aloe juice

METHOD

1 In a blender, combine watermelon, lemon juice, mint, and aloe juice. Purée for 30 seconds or until smooth.

2 Serve immediately, or transfer blending vessel to refrigerator to chill. Blend briefly to recombine ingredients before serving.

NUTRITION PER SERVING	
calories	110
total fat	0g
cholesterol	0mg
sodium	58mg
carbohydrate	29g
dietary fiber	2g
sugars	16g
protein	2g

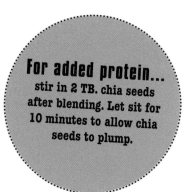

For added protein... stir in 2 TB. chia seeds after blending. Let sit for 10 minutes to allow chia seeds to plump.

Garnish with mint leaves for added digestive benefits.

The vitamin C and antioxidants in lemons help to support a healthy immune system.

For a silkier consistency, replace pineapple with mango.

PINEAPPLE & KALE SOUP

Sweet, juicy pineapple and nutrient-dense kale power this **tropical elixir** that both **refreshes and satisfies.** A touch of **serrano pepper** gives this **transformative soup** just a **hint of heat.** Serve chilled.

PREP & COOK
10 minutes

QUANTITY
Makes 6 cups
Serving size 2 cups

STORAGE
Refrigerated 5 days
Freezing not recommended

INGREDIENTS

2½ cups pineapple, cubed

2½ cups cucumber, chopped

2½ cups coconut water

1¼ cups kale, roughly chopped

¾ cup cilantro, chopped and stems removed

2 tsp. serrano pepper, seeds removed and minced

METHOD

1 In a blender, combine pineapple, cucumber, coconut water, kale, cilantro, and serrano pepper. Purée for 30 seconds or until smooth.

2 Serve immediately, or transfer blending vessel to refrigerator to chill for 30 minutes. Blend briefly before serving to recombine ingredients.

NUTRITION PER SERVING

calories	144
total fat	1g
cholesterol	0mg
sodium	29mg
carbohydrate	35g
dietary fiber	4g
sugars	25g
protein	4g

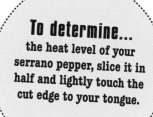

To determine...
the heat level of your serrano pepper, slice it in half and lightly touch the cut edge to your tongue.

Tomatoes are rich in biotin, a B-complex vitamin that helps promote healthy skin.

For a thinner soup, stir in 1 cup tomato juice when adding water.

BELL PEPPER GAZPACHO

The **summer flavors** of **sweet bell pepper** and **cucumber** are highlighted by **red wine vinegar** and **olive oil** in this delicious raw soup. A **tomato base** adds acidity and **rich flavor.** Serve chilled.

PREP & COOK
20 minutes +
24 hours

QUANTITY
Makes 4 cups
Serving size 2 cups

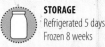

STORAGE
Refrigerated 5 days
Frozen 8 weeks

INGREDIENTS

¾ cup tomatoes, chopped

½ cup red bell pepper, chopped

½ cup yellow bell pepper, chopped

½ cup orange bell pepper, chopped

1 cup cucumber, peeled and chopped

¼ cup red onion, chopped

½ tsp. garlic, minced

¾ cup purified water

1 TB. red wine vinegar

2 TB. extra virgin olive oil

¼ tsp. salt

METHOD

1 In a food processor fitted with a chopping blade, combine tomatoes, red pepper, yellow pepper, orange pepper, cucumber, and red onion. Pulse until ingredients are combined but chunky. (Process in batches if necessary.)

2 Transfer vegetable mixture to a medium nonreactive bowl. Add garlic, water, vinegar, and olive oil. Stir to combine.

3 Refrigerate for 24 hours to allow flavors to meld. Season with salt before serving.

Add...
1 tsp. minced serrano pepper with the other vegetables for a spicy kick and metabolic boost.

NUTRITION PER SERVING

calories	66	carbohydrate	13g
total fat	1g	dietary fiber	4g
cholestoral	0mg	sugars	8g
sodium	301mg	protein	2g

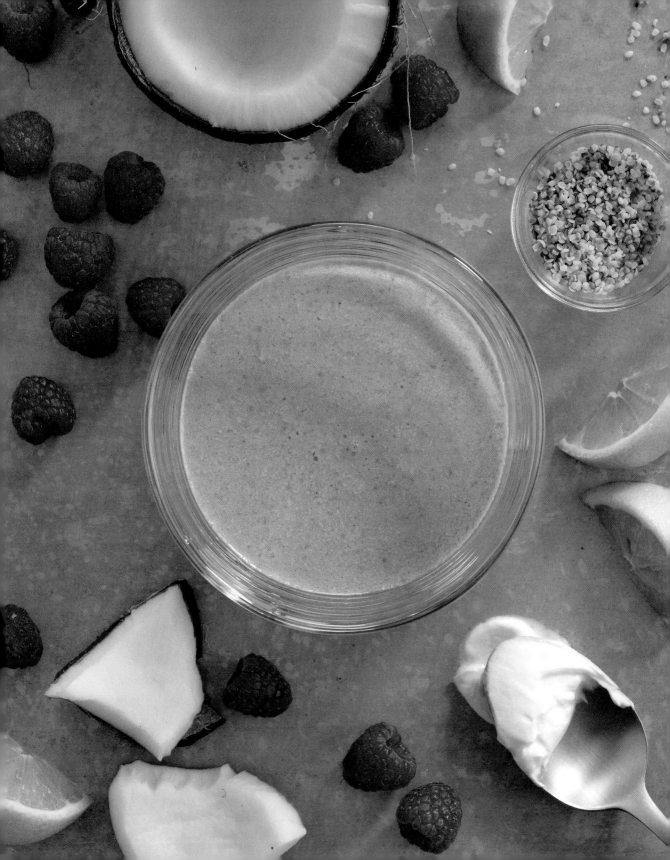

RASPBERRY COCONUT SOUP

With **yogurt and hemp seeds** for protein and fiber, this **tart and creamy** soup is the perfect morning snack. **Sweet raspberries** provide vitamin C, while **coconut flakes** add richness and body. Serve chilled.

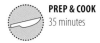 **PREP & COOK**
35 minutes

 QUANTITY
Makes 4 cups
Serving size 1 cup

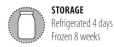 **STORAGE**
Refrigerated 4 days
Frozen 8 weeks

INGREDIENTS

3 cups purified water

1½ cups unsweetened coconut flakes

1½ cups raspberries

4 TB. hemp seeds

½ cup low-fat vanilla yogurt

½ tsp. lemon zest

METHOD

1 In a saucepan over high heat, heat water until just boiling. Remove from heat.

2 In a blender, combine hot water and coconut flakes. Purée for 30 seconds or until smooth. (A high-powered blender is recommended.)

3 Transfer blending vessel to refrigerator for 30 minutes or until well chilled.

4 Once cool, add raspberries, hemp seeds, yogurt, and lemon zest to blender. Purée for 30 seconds.

NUTRITION PER SERVING

calories	253
total fat	20g
cholesterol	2mg
sodium	28mg
carbohydrate	18g
dietary fiber	7g
sugars	8g
protein	7g

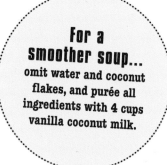
For a smoother soup... omit water and coconut flakes, and purée all ingredients with 4 cups vanilla coconut milk.

4
FALL SOUPING

Fall souping features a beauty boosting cleanse as well as an alkalizing cleanse that will help restore your body to a proper pH balance. The cozy flavors of fall lend rich and creamy textures to recipes that are both comforting and surprisingly healthy.

If butternut squash is not available, try acorn or kabocha squash for a slightly different flavor.

CURRIED BUTTERNUT SOUP

Warming **flavors of curry, ginger,** and **serrano pepper** combine in this creamy autumn soup. Sweet butternut and **rich coconut milk** are balanced with **tart lime juice.** Serve hot.

 PREP & COOK
1 hour

 QUANTITY
Makes 4 cups
Serving size 2 cups

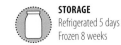 **STORAGE**
Refrigerated 5 days
Frozen 8 weeks

INGREDIENTS

1 small butternut squash, halved and seeds removed

1 TB. olive oil

¾ cup onion, diced

1 clove garlic, minced

1 tsp. serrano pepper, minced

1 (1-in.; 2.5cm) piece fresh ginger, minced

2½ cups purified water

1 tsp. curry powder

Juice of ½ lime

½ cup light coconut milk

1 TB. cilantro, chopped and stems removed

METHOD

1 Preheat oven to 450°F (230°C). Line a baking sheet with foil.

2 Place butternut squash cut side down on prepared baking sheet. Bake for 40 minutes, or until flesh is tender. Scoop the flesh from the skin and measure out 3 cups cooked squash (any extra can be reserved for another purpose).

3 In a medium stockpot, heat oil over medium heat and add onion, garlic, serrano pepper, and ginger. Cook until onions are translucent and garlic is fragrant, about 4 minutes.

4 Add 3 cups cooked butternut squash and water, increase heat, and bring to a boil. Reduce heat and simmer for 15 minutes. Remove from heat.

5 Transfer soup to blender and add curry powder, lime juice, and coconut milk. Purée for 45 seconds or until smooth.

NUTRITION PER SERVING			
calories	251	carbohydrate	41g
total fat	4g	dietary fiber	11g
cholesterol	0mg	sugars	10g
sodium	26mg	protein	4g

Cauliflower is a vitamin C powerhouse and packs a powerful antioxidant punch.

TRUFFLED CAULIFLOWER SOUP

The **velvety texture** of cauliflower and **rich flavor** of truffle oil give this healthy soup an **indulgent** feel. Leeks lend a savory note and deliver **vitamin K** for heart and bone health. Serve hot.

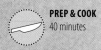 **PREP & COOK**
40 minutes

 QUANTITY
Makes 4 cups
Serving size 2 cups

 STORAGE
Refrigerated 5 days
Frozen 8 weeks

INGREDIENTS

1 TB. coconut oil

2 cups leek, rinsed and diced

2 tsp. garlic, minced (about 2 cloves)

4 cups cauliflower, roughly chopped

5 cups purified water

⅛ tsp. salt

⅛ tsp. pepper

1 tsp. truffle oil

METHOD

1 In a medium stockpot, heat coconut oil over medium heat for 2 minutes. Add leek and garlic and cook until onion is translucent, about 5 minutes.

2 Add cauliflower and water to pot, increase heat, and bring to boil. Reduce heat and simmer for 10 minutes or until cauliflower is cooked through. Remove from heat.

3 Transfer contents of pot to blender. Purée for 30 seconds or until well combined. Season with salt and pepper and blend briefly. Drizzle with truffle oil before serving.

NUTRITION PER SERVING

calories	130
total fat	3g
cholesterol	0mg
sodium	78mg
carbohydrate	23g
dietary fiber	6g
sugars	7g
protein	5g

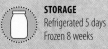

For a more... complex flavor, add a Parmesan rind to the pot while cauliflower cooks. Remove prior to blending, and finish soup with a sprinkling of chopped chives.

Almonds are alkalizing, aid in brain function, and provide satiety.

Coconut is high in phosphorus, which helps strengthen teeth and bones

ALMOND CACAO SOUP

Rich and satisfying, this **dessert soup** is full of **chocolatey, nutty flavor**. With healthy fats and protein from **almonds, hemp seeds, and coconut**, it's **a treat you can feel good about**. Serve chilled.

 PREP & COOK
35 minutes

 QUANTITY
Makes 4 cups
Serving size 1 cup

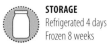 **STORAGE**
Refrigerated 4 days
Frozen 8 weeks

INGREDIENTS

1 cup raw almonds

2 cups purified water

1 cup coconut water

3 TB. cacao nibs

1 TB. agave nectar

1 TB. unsweetened coconut flakes

4 TB. hemp seeds

METHOD

1 Place almonds in medium bowl and cover with boiling water. Let sit for at least 30 minutes to soften. Drain almonds and discard soaking water.

2 In a blender, combine almonds and 2 cups water. Blend for 30 seconds or until no chunks of almond remain and you are left with a creamy milk.

3 Add coconut water, cacao nibs, agave nectar, coconut flakes, and hemp seeds. Blend for 30 seconds or until cacao is completely broken down and incorporated.

NUTRITION PER SERVING

calories	299
total fat	24g
cholesterol	0mg
sodium	15mg
carbohydrate	16g
dietary fiber	5g
sugars	8g
protein	11g

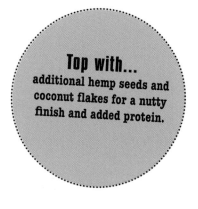

Top with...
additional hemp seeds and coconut flakes for a nutty finish and added protein.

GINGER SWEET POTATO SOUP

Sweet and spicy, this satisfying soup features nutrient-dense sweet potatoes, **rejuvenating ginger,** and **earthy turmeric.** With high levels of **immune-boosting vitamin C,** it's perfect for cold season. Serve hot.

 PREP & COOK
30 minutes

 QUANTITY
Makes 3 cups
Serving size 2 cups

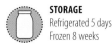 **STORAGE**
Refrigerated 5 days
Frozen 8 weeks

INGREDIENTS

¾ TB. coconut oil

¾ cup onion, diced

½ TB. garlic, minced

1½ cups sweet potato, peeled and diced

½ cup carrot, peeled and diced

2 cups purified water

1½ TB. coconut milk

1 (1-in.; 2.5cm) piece fresh ginger, grated

1 (1-in.; 2.5cm) piece turmeric root, grated

½ TB. chives, chopped

¼ tsp. salt

⅛ tsp. pepper

METHOD

1 In a medium stockpot, heat coconut oil over medium heat for 2 minutes. Add onion and garlic and cook until onion is translucent, about 5 minutes.

2 Add sweet potoato, carrot, and water. Increase heat and bring to a boil. Reduce heat and simmer for 10 minutes or until vegetables are cooked through. Remove from heat.

3 Transfer contents of pot to blender. Add coconut milk, ginger, and turmeric, and purée until smooth. Add chives, salt, and pepper, and blend briefly before serving.

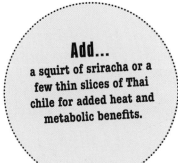

Add...
a squirt of sriracha or a few thin slices of Thai chile for added heat and metabolic benefits.

NUTRITION PER SERVING	
calories	174
total fat	4g
cholesterol	0mg
sodium	374mg
carbohydrate	32g
dietary fiber	6g
sugars	9g
protein	3g

Sweet potato can be replaced with butternut squash or additional carrot, if desired.

ALKALIZE
3-DAY CLEANSE

The pH of the body is directly affected by what you consume each day. A diet high in processed foods, meat, dairy, and grains causes the body to become acidic and drop below the optimal pH level of 7.4. When the pH level drops, your body is more susceptible to disease and illness. This cleanse will help restore the body's natural alkaline state.

Follow for 3 days for optimal benefits.

Shopping List

Fridge/Freezer

Garlic (8 cloves)

Onions (6)

Asparagus (1 bunch)

Baby spinach (5 cups)

Romaine lettuce (4 cups)

Kale (1¼ cups, chopped)

Fresh ginger (1 [1-in.; 2.5cm] piece)

Fresh sweet corn (6 ears)

Cucumber (2 medium)

Serrano pepper (1)

Lemons (4)

Watermelon (3 cups, cubed)

Pineapple (2½ cups, cubed)

Mint (3 TB., chopped)

Cilantro (1 bunch)

Chives (4 TB., chopped)

Pantry

Olive oil (3 TB.)

Coconut oil (2 TB.)

Aloe juice (4 cups)

Coconut water (2½ cups)

Light coconut milk (¼ cup)

Purified water (4 qt.; 4l)

Cashews, unsalted (1 cup)

Agave nectar (1 tsp.)

Dried figs (¼ cup)

Quinoa, uncooked (½ cup)

Cardamom pods (8–10)

Vanilla bean (1)

Salt

Pepper

PREPARATION			DURING THE CLEANSE	
1 WEEK BEFORE	**3 DAYS BEFORE**	**1 DAY BEFORE**	**DAILY SOUPS**	**CLEANSE BOOSTERS**
★ Make **Sweet Corn & Chive Soup** (single batch); freeze in 2-cup portions. RECIPE PAGE 69	★ Make **Ginger Greens Soup** (double batch); refrigerate in 2-cup portions. RECIPE PAGE 48	★ Make **Watermelon Aloe Mint Soup** (single batch); refrigerate in 2-cup portions. RECIPE PAGE 80	**BREAKFAST** Watermelon Aloe Mint Soup (2 cups)	★ Drink 2 cups of alkalized water between meals.
★ Make **Asparagus Soup with Mint** (double batch); freeze in 2-cup portions. RECIPE PAGE 51	★ Make **Pineapple & Kale Soup** (single batch); refrigerate in 2-cup portions. RECIPE PAGE 83	★ Make **Fig & Cardamom Soup** (single batch); refrigerate in 1-cup portions. RECIPE PAGE 126	**SNACK** Sweet Corn & Chive Soup (2 cups) **LUNCH** Ginger Greens Soup (2 cups)	★ Perform 30 to 60 minutes of light to moderate exercise daily during cleanse. Focus on yoga or other mind-body exercises in particular, as stress can also cause acidity to build in the body.
★ Eliminate processed foods and sugar from your diet and focus on whole foods.	★ Eliminate poultry, meat, and dairy from your diet. ★ Focus on vegetable-based meals supplemented with fish, grains, and legumes. ★ Drink at least 8 cups of water.	★ Transfer Sweet Corn & Chive Soup and Asparagus Soup with Mint from freezer to refrigerator to thaw. ★ Eliminate all animal products from your diet. ★ Eat vegetable-based meals with some legumes, grains, and nuts. ★ Drink at least 8 cups of water.	**SNACK** Pineapple & Kale Soup (2 cups) **DINNER** Asparagus Soup with Mint (2 cups) **DESSERT** Fig & Cardamom Soup (1 cup) **ALTERNATIVES** Mango Soup with Lime (breakfast) RECIPE PAGE 27 Carrot & Fennel Soup (dinner) RECIPE PAGE 146	

APPLE & AMARANTH SOUP

Sweet and luxurious, this is the perfect soup for a chilly autumn morning. **Protein-rich amaranth** forms a filling base, while **warming cinnamon** adds a spicy note. Serve hot.

 PREP & COOK
25 minutes

 QUANTITY
Makes 5 cups
Serving size 2 cups

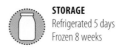 **STORAGE**
Refrigerated 5 days
Frozen 8 weeks

INGREDIENTS

4 cups Fuji apples, peeled and diced

4 cups purified water

3 cinnamon sticks

½ cup amaranth, cooked

METHOD

1 In a medium stockpot, combine apples, water, and cinnamon sticks. Bring to a boil over high heat, and then reduce to a simmer and cover. Cook for 20 minutes or until apples are cooked through.

2 Remove cinnamon sticks and transfer contents of pot to blender. Add amaranth and blend until smooth. Add water if needed to thin.

NUTRITION PER SERVING

calories	168
total fat	1g
cholesterol	0mg
sodium	4mg
carbohydrate	40g
dietary fiber	4g
sugars	22g
protein	3g

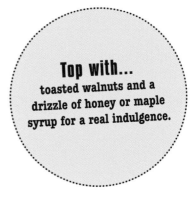
Top with...
toasted walnuts and a drizzle of honey or maple syrup for a real indulgence.

Amaranth is high in fiber and an excellent source of protein.

BLACK BEAN POBLANO SOUP

Protein-rich black beans are the foundation of this **hearty, spicy soup,** which is seasoned with **garlic** and **cumin.** Poblano peppers, along with **three types of chile powder,** add heat and flavor. Serve hot.

 PREP & COOK
50 minutes

 QUANTITY
Makes 4 cups
Serving size 2 cups

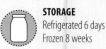 **STORAGE**
Refrigerated 6 days
Frozen 8 weeks

INGREDIENTS

2 TB. olive oil

⅓ cup onion, diced

⅓ cup carrot, diced

⅓ cup celery, diced

½ cup poblano pepper, diced

1 TB. garlic, minced (about 3 cloves)

1 TB. tomato paste

1 (14.5-oz.; 411g) can diced tomatoes

1 (15-oz.; 425g) can black beans, drained and rinsed

1 tsp. chile de árbol

1 TB. ground cumin

1 TB. ancho chile powder (optional)

½ TB. chili powder

½ tsp. salt

6 cups purified water

Juice of 1 lime

2 TB. cilantro, minced

METHOD

1 In a stockpot, heat olive oil over medium heat. Add onion, carrot, celery, poblano pepper, and garlic. Cook until onions are translucent, about 5 minutes. Add tomato paste and toss to coat. Cook for another 5 minutes.

2 Add diced tomatoes (with liquid), black beans, chile de árbol, cumin, ancho chile powder (if using), chili powder, salt, and water. Increase heat and bring to boil, then reduce heat and simmer for 20 minutes or until water has slightly reduced and vegetables are tender.

3 Carefully transfer contents of pot to blender and add lime juice and cilantro. Purée until smooth, about 45 seconds.

NUTRITION PER SERVING

calories	262
total fat	4g
cholesterol	0mg
sodium	1,727mg
carbohydrate	48g
dietary fiber	21g
sugars	7g
protein	15g

SQUASH & CRANBERRY SOUP

Sweet and savory, this satisfying soup features **roasted acorn squash** and **tart cranberries** accented with the **autumn flavors of ginger, rosemary,** and **maple syrup.** Serve hot.

PREP & COOK
50 minutes

QUANTITY
Makes 4 cups
Serving size 2 cups

STORAGE
Refrigerated 5 days
Frozen 8 weeks

INGREDIENTS

2 acorn squash, halved and seeds removed

2 TB. olive oil

1½ cups onion, diced

1½ tsp. garlic, minced

2 cinnamon sticks

4½ cups purified water

1 cup cranberries

2 TB. pure maple syrup

2 tsp. fresh ginger, grated

1 tsp. fresh rosemary, minced

¼ tsp. salt

¼ tsp. pepper

METHOD

1 Preheat oven to 425°F (220°C). Line a baking sheet with foil. Place squash cut side down on prepared baking sheet. Bake for 15 minutes. Scoop flesh from skin and measure 4 cups cooked squash (any extra squash can be saved for later use).

2 In a medium stockpot, heat olive oil over medium heat for 2 minutes. Add onion and garlic and cook until onion is translucent, about 5 minutes.

3 Add water, 4 cups cooked squash, and cinnamon sticks. Increase heat and bring to a boil, then reduce heat and cover. Simmer for 20 minutes. Add cranberries and simmer for another 5 minutes. Remove from heat.

4 Remove cinnamon sticks and carefully transfer contents of pot to blender. Blend until soup is smooth and ingredients are well combined. Add maple syrup, ginger, and rosemary and blend briefly. Season with salt and pepper before serving.

NUTRITION PER SERVING

calories	262
total fat	2g
cholesterol	0mg
sodium	308mg
carbohydrate	63g
dietary fiber	9g
sugars	20g
protein	4g

FENNEL & TOMATO SOUP

This **rich, savory soup** combines **umami-rich tomatoes** with aromatic fennel and **sweet carrots** to create a **hearty, warming meal** that can be enjoyed for lunch or dinner. Serve hot.

 PREP & COOK
40 minutes

 QUANTITY
Makes 3 cups
Serving size 2 cups

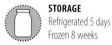 **STORAGE**
Refrigerated 5 days
Frozen 8 weeks

INGREDIENTS

1 TB. olive oil

¾ cup onion, diced

2 tsp. garlic, minced (about 2 cloves)

2 cups fennel, diced

¼ tsp. fennel seeds

⅓ cup carrot, diced

2 cups tomato, diced

2 cups purified water

¼ tsp. salt

⅛ tsp. pepper

METHOD

1 In a medium stockpot, heat olive oil over medium heat. Add onion and garlic and cook until onion is translucent and garlic is fragrant, about 4 minutes.

2 Add fennel, fennel seeds, and carrot, and cook until fennel is fragrant, about 2 minutes.

3 Add tomatoes and water, increase heat, and bring to a boil. Reduce heat and simmer for 20 minutes.

4 Carefully transfer contents of pot to blender. Purée until smooth, about 30 seconds. Taste and season with salt and pepper, and blend briefly to combine.

NUTRITION PER SERVING

calories	167
total fat	8g
cholesterol	9mg
sodium	360mg
carbohydrate	17g
dietary fiber	6g
sugars	9g
protein	4g

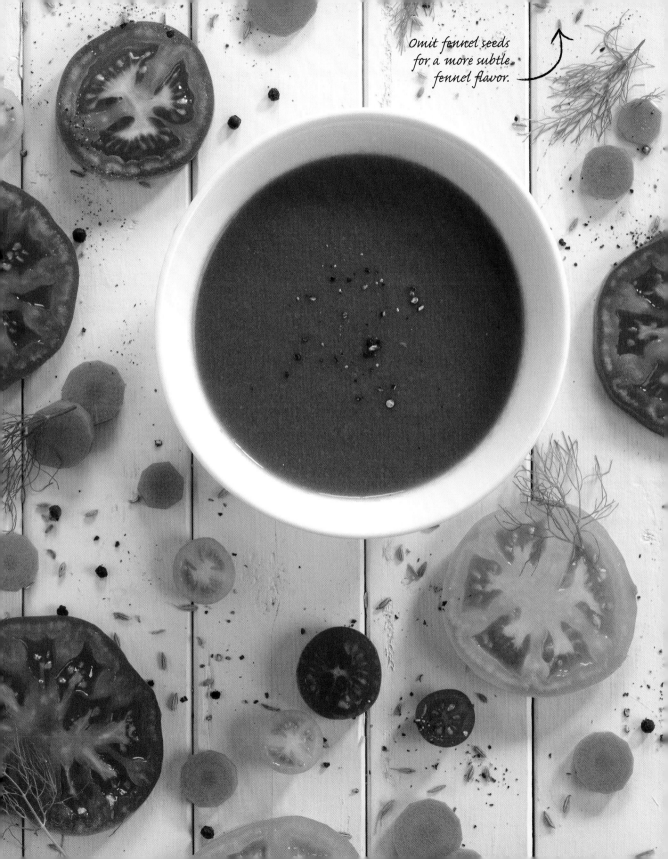

Omit fennel seeds for a more subtle fennel flavor.

APPLE & PARSNIP SOUP

Earthy, slightly **sweet parsnips** pair perfectly with **tart apples** in this smooth, **comforting soup**. Warm, **cozy vanilla** and a **hint of cinnamon** add **aroma and spice**. Serve hot.

PREP & COOK
35 minutes

QUANTITY
Makes 4 cups
Serving size 1 cup

STORAGE
Refrigerated 5 days
Frozen 8 weeks

INGREDIENTS

1 TB. coconut oil

¾ cup onion, diced

1½ cups parsnip, peeled and diced

1 cinnamon stick

3 cups Granny Smith apple, peeled and diced

4 cups purified water

¾ TB. vanilla extract, or seeds from 1 vanilla bean

⅛ tsp. salt

METHOD

1 In a medium stockpot, heat coconut oil over medium heat for 2 minutes. Add onion and cook until translucent, about 5 minutes.

2 Add parsnips and water to pot. Bring to a boil, reduce heat, and simmer for 5 minutes.

3 Add cinnamon stick and apples, return to a boil, and then reduce heat to simmer until apples and parsnips are cooked through, about 10 minutes.

4 Remove cinnamon stick and discard. Carefully transfer contents of pot to blender and add vanilla. Purée until smooth, about 30 seconds. Season with salt.

NUTRITION PER SERVING	
calories	204
total fat	2g
cholesterol	0mg
sodium	158mg
carbohydrate	45g
dietary fiber	8g
sugars	25g
protein	2g

BANANA WALNUT SOUP

This **sweet and creamy soup** is rich in the natural sleep-aid melatonin, making it a **perfect bedtime snack.** Heat-healthy **walnuts** and **flax seeds** add richness along with **omega-3s.** Serve chilled.

 PREP & COOK
12 hours

 QUANTITY
Makes 4 cups
Serving size 1 cup

STORAGE
Refrigerated 5 days
Freezing not recommended

INGREDIENTS

3 cups purified water

1 cup walnuts

1 cinnamon stick

2 bananas, peeled and cut into large chunks

½ tsp. vanilla extract, or seeds from ½ vanilla bean

2 tsp. ground flax seed

METHOD

1 In a saucepan over high heat, bring water to a boil. Place walnuts and cinnamon stick in a heat-tolerant bowl and cover with boiling water. Let cool and refrigerate overnight.

2 Remove cinnamon stick and transfer walnuts and soaking water to blender. Add bananas, vanilla, and flax seed. Purée until smooth, about 30 seconds.

NUTRITION PER SERVING	
calories	273
total fat	21g
cholesterol	0mg
sodium	2mg
carbohydrate	20g
dietary fiber	4g
sugars	10g
protein	6g

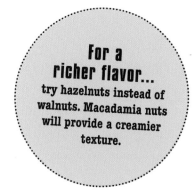

For a richer flavor... try hazelnuts instead of walnuts. Macadamia nuts will provide a creamier texture.

Fresh chives are a
good source of folate.

Apples are rich in vitamin C and
an excellent source of fiber.

APPLE & CELERIAC SOUP

Humble celeriac is elevated when paired with **crisp apples** and **savory onions** to make a **silky, distinctively delicious soup.** Mild and soothing, it's a comforting meal for fall. Serve hot.

PREP & COOK
30 minutes

QUANTITY
Makes 2 cups
Serving size 2 cups

STORAGE
Refrigerated 5 days
Frozen 8 weeks

INGREDIENTS

1 tsp. coconut oil

½ cup onion, diced

½ tsp. garlic, minced

1 cup Granny Smith apple, peeled and diced

1 cup celeriac, peeled and diced

2 cups purified water

2 TB. chives, chopped

⅛ tsp. salt

METHOD

1 In a medium stockpot, heat coconut oil over medium heat for 2 minutes. Add onion and garlic and cook until onion is translucent, about 5 minutes.

2 Add apple, celeriac, and water. Increase heat and bring to a boil, and then reduce simmer for 12 minutes or until apple and celeriac are cooked through. Remove from heat.

3 Transfer contents of pot to blender. Carefully purée until smooth, about 30 seconds. Stir in chives before serving.

NUTRITION PER SERVING

calories	255
total fat	5g
cholesterol	0mg
sodium	450mg
carbohydrate	53g
dietary fiber	9g
sugars	29g
protein	4g

To make...
Spicy Apple Celeriac Soup, omit chives and add 1 tsp. minced serrano pepper, 1 tsp. grated fresh ginger, and a squeeze of lime juice.

BEAUTY REBOOT
3-DAY CLEANSE

Your diet plays a role in how you look as well as how you feel. A diet high in processed foods, sugar, refined carbohydrates, and little water can result in dull skin, dry hair, and brittle nails. Hydrating, nutrient-dense soups can help correct these issues and give your appearance a boost.

Follow for 3 days to nourish skin, hair, and nails. For a quick pick-me-up, do a 1-day cleanse program.

Shopping List

Fridge/Freezer

Onions (6)
Carrots (10 medium)
Celery (3 stalks)
Rhubarb (²/₃ cup, diced)
Garlic (12 cloves)
Avocado (1)
Fennel (2 bulbs)
Cucumbers (2)
Arugula (2 cups)
Butter lettuce (2 cups, chopped)
Lemon (1)
Peaches (5)
Strawberries (2 cups)
Parsley (1 bunch)
Fresh basil (¾ cup, chopped)
Fresh thyme (1 tsp., minced)
Cilantro (½ cup, chopped)
Ginger (4 TB., grated)
Beef bones (4 lb.; 2kg)

Pantry

Olive oil (7 TB.)
Coconut oil (4 TB.)
Apple cider vinegar (2 TB.)
Red wine vinegar (3 TB.)
Fire-roasted diced tomatoes (1 cup)
Roasted red pepper (3 cups)
Chickpeas, canned (1 cup)
Tomato paste (3 TB.)
Macadamia nuts (¾ cup)
Honey (4 TB.)
Agave nectar (2 TB.)
Coconut water (3 cups)
Purified water (9 qt.; 9l)
Bay leaf (1)
Red pepper flakes (½ tsp.)
Salt
Pepper

PREPARATION			DURING THE CLEANSE	
1 WEEK BEFORE	**2 DAYS BEFORE**	**1 DAY BEFORE**	**DAILY SOUPS**	**CLEANSE BOOSTERS**
★ Make **Ginger Beef Bone Broth** (single batch); freeze in 2-cup portions. RECIPE PAGE 166	★ Make **Peach Soup with Basil** (single batch); refrigerate in 2-cup portions. RECIPE PAGE 70	★ Make **Avocado & Arugula Soup** (double batch); refrigerate in 2-cup portions. RECIPE PAGE 29	**BREAKFAST** Peach Soup with Basil (2 cups)	★ Drink 2 cups of alkalized water between meals.
★ Make **Red Pepper Chickpea Soup** (double batch); freeze in 2-cup portions. RECIPE PAGE 138	★ Make **Carrot & Fennel Soup** (double batch); refrigerate in 2-cup portions. RECIPE PAGE 146	★ Make **Strawberry Rhubarb Soup** (single batch); refrigerate in 1-cup portions. RECIPE PAGE 54	**SNACK** Ginger Beef Bone Broth (2 cups) **LUNCH** Avocado & Arugula Soup (2 cups)	★ Perform 30 to 60 minutes of light to moderate exercise daily during cleanse, particularly hot yoga to aid in detoxification.
★ Eliminate processed foods and sugar from your diet and focus on whole foods.	★ Transfer Ginger Beef Bone Broth and Red Pepper Chickpea Soup from freezer to refrigerator to thaw.	★ Eliminate all animal products from your diet.	**SNACK** Carrot & Fennel Soup (2 cups) **DINNER** Red Pepper Chickpea Soup (2 cups)	★ Receive a colonic treatment halfway through or at the end of your cleanse.
	★ Eliminate poultry, meat, and dairy from your diet.	★ Eat vegetable-based meals with some legumes, grains, and nuts.	**DESSERT** Strawberry Rhubarb Soup (1 cup)	
	★ Focus on vegetable-based meals supplemented with fish, grains, and legumes.	★ Drink at least 8 cups of water.	**ALTERNATIVES** Kiwi Kale Gazpacho (lunch) RECIPE PAGE 36 Leafy Greens Detox Soup (dinner) RECIPE PAGE 116	

Celery contains vitamin C, which has excellent antioxidant properties.

The lentils in this soup are high in fiber and rich in copper, which is important for bone strength and tissue health.

FRENCH LENTIL SOUP

Simple but immensely satisfying, this recipe allows the ingredients to shine. **Earthy lentils, sweet carrots,** and **savory leeks** combine in a **rustic soup** that's hearty and filling. Serve hot.

PREP & COOK
40 minutes

QUANTITY
Makes 4 cups
Serving size 2 cups

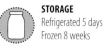

STORAGE
Refrigerated 5 days
Frozen 8 weeks

INGREDIENTS

1 TB. olive oil

1 cup leeks, rinsed
and diced

1 cup carrot, peeled
and diced

1 cup celery, diced

1½ TB. garlic, minced

1 cup French green lentils,
uncooked

6 cups purified water

¼ tsp. salt

⅛ tsp. pepper

METHOD

1 In a medium stockpot, heat olive oil over medium heat for 2 minutes. Add leeks, carrots, celery, and garlic and cook until leeks are translucent, about 5 minutes.

2 Add lentils and water, increase heat, and bring to a boil. Reduce heat, cover, and simmer for 20 minutes or until lentils are fully cooked. Season with salt and pepper.

NUTRITION PER SERVING

calories	420
total fat	3g
cholesterol	0mg
sodium	390mg
carbohydrate	77g
dietary fiber	14g
sugars	7g
protein	26g

For an added...
health boost, use beef bone broth instead of water and finish with a touch of fresh grated turmeric.

GRAPEFRUIT & FENNEL SOUP

This **refreshing, herbaceous blend** features the **tart, tangy flavor** of grapefruit along with **lightly sweet, earthy fennel.** Spinach adds a **vegetal note** as well as **antioxidant benefits.** Serve chilled.

PREP & COOK
15 minutes

QUANTITY
Makes 4 cups
Serving size 2 cups

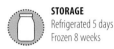

STORAGE
Refrigerated 5 days
Frozen 8 weeks

INGREDIENTS

2 cups fresh-squeezed grapefruit juice (about 6 grapefruits)

1 cup coconut water

1 cup fennel, bulb and fronds, chopped

1 cup baby spinach

2 tsp. agave nectar

METHOD

1 In a blender, combine grapefruit juice, coconut water, fennel, spinach, and agave nectar. Purée until mixture is smooth and fennel is completely incorporated.

2 If desired, transfer blending vessel to refrigerator to chill for 30 minutes. Blend briefly to recombine ingredients before serving.

NUTRITION PER SERVING

calories	192
total fat	2g
cholesterol	0mg
sodium	162mg
carbohydrate	40g
dietary fiber	6g
sugars	8g
protein	4g

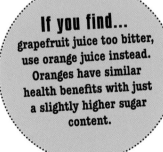

If you find...
grapefruit juice too bitter, use orange juice instead. Oranges have similar health benefits with just a slightly higher sugar content.

Grapefruit is rich in vitamin C and lycopene, a compound with powerful antioxidant properties.

LEAFY GREENS DETOX SOUP

Carrot, onion, and celery soften the bitterness of **kale and spinach** in this **verdant, detoxifying medley.** The hearty greens are **brightened by lemon juice** and a dash of red pepper flakes. Serve hot.

 PREP & COOK
40 minutes

 QUANTITY
Makes 4 cups
Serving size 2 cups

 STORAGE
Refrigerated 5 days
Frozen 8 weeks

INGREDIENTS

2 TB. coconut oil

1½ cups onion, diced

1½ cups carrot, peeled and diced

1½ cups celery, diced

2 tsp. garlic, minced (about 2 cloves)

4½ cups purified water

2 cups kale, stems removed and roughly chopped

4 cups baby spinach, tightly packed

½ tsp. red pepper flakes

2 TB. lemon juice

½ tsp. salt

METHOD

1 In a medium stockpot, heat coconut oil over medium heat for 2 minutes. Add onion, carrot, celery, and garlic and cook until onion is translucent, about 5 minutes.

2 Add water, increase heat, and bring to a boil. Then reduce heat and simmer for 20 minutes or until vegetables are cooked through. Remove from heat. Stir in kale, spinach, red pepper flakes, lemon juice, and salt.

3 Transfer contents of pot to blender and carefully purée until smooth and well combined. Add water if needed to thin.

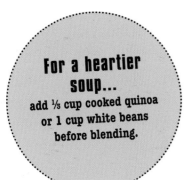

For a heartier soup...
add ⅓ cup cooked quinoa or 1 cup white beans before blending.

NUTRITION PER SERVING	
calories	146
total fat	2g
cholesterol	0mg
sodium	476mg
carbohydrate	30g
dietary fiber	8g
sugars	12g
protein	5g

The vitamins and minerals in dark, leafy greens improve blood flow, purify the blood, and boost immunity

Pears are high in fiber and rich in copper, which plays an important role in energy production.

PEAR SOUP WITH CINNAMON

The **subtle, sweet flavor of pear** shines when combined with **juicy apples** and highlighted by **spicy cinnamon** and **fresh-grated nutmeg** in this **warm, comforting soup.** Serve hot.

PREP & COOK
20 minutes

QUANTITY
Makes 4 cups
Serving size 2 cups

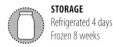
STORAGE
Refrigerated 4 days
Frozen 8 weeks

INGREDIENTS

4 pears, peeled and cubed
2 apples, peeled and cubed
2 cinnamon sticks
2 cups purified water
1 TB. palm sugar
¼ tsp. fresh nutmeg, grated

METHOD

1 In a medium stockpot, combine pears, apples, cinnamon sticks, and water. Bring to a boil over high heat, and then reduce heat and simmer for 10 minutes or until fruit is cooked through.

2 Remove cinnamon sticks and transfer contents of pot to blender. Add sugar and grated nutmeg. Purée until smooth. Taste and adjust sugar based on sweetness of fruit.

NUTRITION PER SERVING

calories	266
total fat	1g
cholesterol	0mg
sodium	3mg
carbohydrate	70g
dietary fiber	12g
sugars	49g
protein	2g

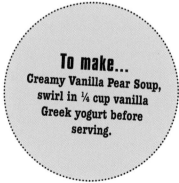
To make...
Creamy Vanilla Pear Soup, swirl in ¼ cup vanilla Greek yogurt before serving.

SPICY LEMONGRASS SOUP

This **soothing, aromatic soup** contains **lemongrass and ginger** to aid in digestion and bok choy to **reduce inflammation.** Chili paste adds a **spicy note** as well as a **metabolic boost.** Serve hot.

PREP & COOK
40 minutes

QUANTITY
Makes 4 cups
Serving size 2 cups

STORAGE
Refrigerated 5 days
Frozen 8 weeks

INGREDIENTS

¾ TB. coconut oil

1 cup onion, diced

2 stalks lemongrass, cut into 2-inch (5cm) pieces

1½ tsp. garlic, minced

¾ cup carrot, peeled and cut into rounds

1 (5-in; 12.5cm) piece fresh ginger, peeled and cut into chunks

1 TB. chili paste

4½ cups purified water

2 cups bok choy, roughly chopped

2 TB. green onion, sliced

2 TB. cilantro, stems removed and minced

Juice of 1 lime

½ tsp. salt

METHOD

1 In a medium stockpot, heat coconut oil over medium heat for 2 minutes. Add onion, lemongrass, garlic, carrot, and ginger. Cook for 5 minutes or until onion is translucent and garlic is fragrant.

2 Add chili paste and continue to cook for another 2 minutes, stirring to combine.

3 Add water, increase heat, and bring to a boil. Then reduce heat, cover, and simmer for 20 minutes.

4 With a sieve or slotted spoon, remove lemongrass and ginger. Add bok choy and simmer for 3 minutes or until it is cooked through.

5 Remove from heat. Stir in green onion, cilantro, lime juice, and salt.

NUTRITION PER SERVING

calories	121	carbohydrate	24g
total fat	2g	dietary fiber	7g
cholestoral	0g	sugars	8g
sodium	112mg	protein	5g

SPLIT PEA SOUP WITH KALE

Creamy and **packed with nutrition,** this hearty pea soup **flecked with kale** makes a satisfying meal on a chilly day. **Full of protein** and fiber, it's **comfort food** at its best. Serve hot.

PREP & COOK
40 minutes

QUANTITY
Makes 4 cups
Serving size 2 cups

STORAGE
Refrigerated 4 days
Frozen 8 weeks

INGREDIENTS

¾ TB. olive oil

½ cup carrot, peeled and diced

½ cup celery, diced

½ cup onion, diced

1 TB. garlic, minced (about 3 cloves)

5 cups purified water

1 cup split peas (uncooked)

½ cup kale, deveined and minced

1 tsp. salt

⅛ tsp. pepper

METHOD

1 In a medium stockpot, heat olive oil over medium heat for 2 minutes. Add carrot, celery, onion, and garlic. Cook for 5 minutes or until onion is translucent.

2 Add water and split peas, increase heat, and bring to a boil. Reduce heat, cover, and simmer for 25 minutes or until peas have completely softened.

3 Stir in kale and cook until wilted, about 3 minutes. Season with salt and pepper. If desired, use an immersion blender to purée to a smooth consistency.

NUTRITION PER SERVING

calories	184
total fat	4g
cholesterol	0mg
sodium	1,428mg
carbohydrate	30g
dietary fiber	10g
sugars	6g
protein	10g

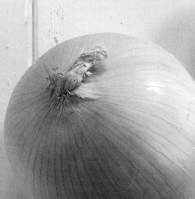

5
WINTER SOUPING

Winter souping features a detoxifying cleanse as well as an immunity-boosting cleanse that will help stave off winter's bite. Root vegetables are the stars in these heartier recipes that not only nourish, but help to energize the body during cold winter months.

Mushrooms are one of the few food sources of vitamin D, and the only vegan source.

MUSHROOM & FREEKEH SOUP

High in protein with a **creamy texture,** this hearty combination of mushrooms, parsley, rosemary, and the **supergrain freekeh** is a **rich, satisfying** source of energy. Serve hot.

 PREP & COOK
55 minutes

 QUANTITY
Makes 4 cups
Serving size 2 cups

 STORAGE
Refrigerated 5 days
Frozen 8 weeks

INGREDIENTS

2 TB. olive oil

½ cup leeks, rinsed and diced

½ cup carrot, peeled and diced

½ cup celery, diced

¾ TB. garlic, minced

½ TB. tomato paste

1 cup shiitake mushroom, diced

1 cup cremini mushroom, diced

3 cups purified water

¾ cup freekeh, cooked

2 TB. parsley, minced

½ tsp. fresh rosemary, minced

½ tsp. salt

¼ tsp. pepper

METHOD

1 In a medium stock pot, heat olive oil over medium heat for 2 minutes. Add leeks, carrot, celery, and garlic, and cook until leeks are translucent, about 5 minutes.

2 Add tomato paste and continue to cook vegetables for another 5 minutes. Add mushrooms and water. Increase heat and bring to a boil, and then reduce heat and simmer for 10 minutes or until mushrooms are cooked through.

3 Transfer contents of pot to blender and add freekeh. Blend until smooth, adding water to thin if needed. Add parsley, rosemary, salt, and pepper and blend briefly to combine.

NUTRITION PER SERVING	
calories	225
total fat	15g
cholesterol	0mg
sodium	648mg
carbohydrate	21g
dietary fiber	6g
sugars	4g
protein	5g

FIG & CARDAMOM SOUP

The **sweet flavor of dried figs** and **rich nuttiness of cashews** are accented with **floral notes of cardamom** in this protein-rich soup. It's a **satisfying morning meal** or energizing afternoon snack. Serve chilled.

 PREP & COOK
45 minutes

 QUANTITY
Makes 3 cups
Serving size 1 cup

 STORAGE
Refrigerated 5 days
Frozen 8 weeks

INGREDIENTS

2 cups purified water

1 cup unsalted cashews

1 cup quinoa, cooked

½ tsp. cardamom seeds
    (from 8–10 pods)

Seeds of 1 vanilla bean pod

1 tsp. agave nectar

¼ cup dried figs, stems
    removed and quartered

METHOD

1 In a small saucepan, heat water until just boiling. Place cashews in a medium, heat-safe bowl and add boiling water to cover. Let sit for 10 minutes.

2 Transfer cashews and soaking water to a blender. Purée for 30 seconds or until smooth.

3 Using a mortar and pestle, grind cardamom seeds to a fine powder. Add quinoa, ground cardamom seeds, vanilla bean seeds, agave nectar, and dried figs to blender with processed cashews. Purée until smooth.

4 Transfer blending vessel to refrigerator to chill for 30 minutes. Blend briefly to recombine ingredients before serving. Add water or cashew milk to thin, if needed.

NUTRITION PER SERVING

calories	335
total fat	19g
cholesterol	0mg
sodium	3mg
carbohydrate	39g
dietary fiber	5g
sugars	9g
protein	11g

If you are...
unable to find cardamom,
or feel the flavor is too
intense, use a more subtle
spice, like ginger, instead.

Heart-healthy figs are loaded with fiber and potassium, which helps regulate blood pressure.

Zucchini is a good source
of potassium, which
helps maintain normal
blood pressure and
healthy kidneys.

FENNEL & ZUCCHINI SOUP

Zucchini brings a **velvety texture** and mild flavor to this **delicate soup,** allowing the **anise notes of fennel** to shine. Onion and garlic provide a **savory balance** and depth of flavor. Serve hot.

PREP & COOK
20 minutes

QUANTITY
Makes 4 cups
Serving size 2 cups

STORAGE
Refrigerated 5 days
Frozen 8 weeks

INGREDIENTS

1 TB. coconut oil

1 cup onion, diced

3 cups fennel, bulb and
  fronds, diced

¾ tsp. garlic

2 cups zucchini, diced

4¼ cups purified water

⅛ tsp. salt

⅛ tsp. pepper

METHOD

1 In a medium stockpot, heat coconut oil over medium heat for 2 minutes. Add onion, fennel, and garlic and cook until onion is translucent, about 5 minutes.

2 Add zucchini and water. Increase heat and bring to a boil, then reduce and simmer for 7 minutes or until vegetables are cooked through. Remove from heat.

3 Transfer contents of pot to blender. Season with salt and pepper and purée until smooth.

NUTRITION PER SERVING

calories	113
total fat	2g
cholesterol	0mg
sodium	222mg
carbohydrate	22g
dietary fiber	7g
sugars	12g
protein	5g

To make...
Sweet Fennel & Pear Soup,
omit garlic, salt, and
pepper, and replace the
zucchini with 2 cups
chopped and peeled pear.

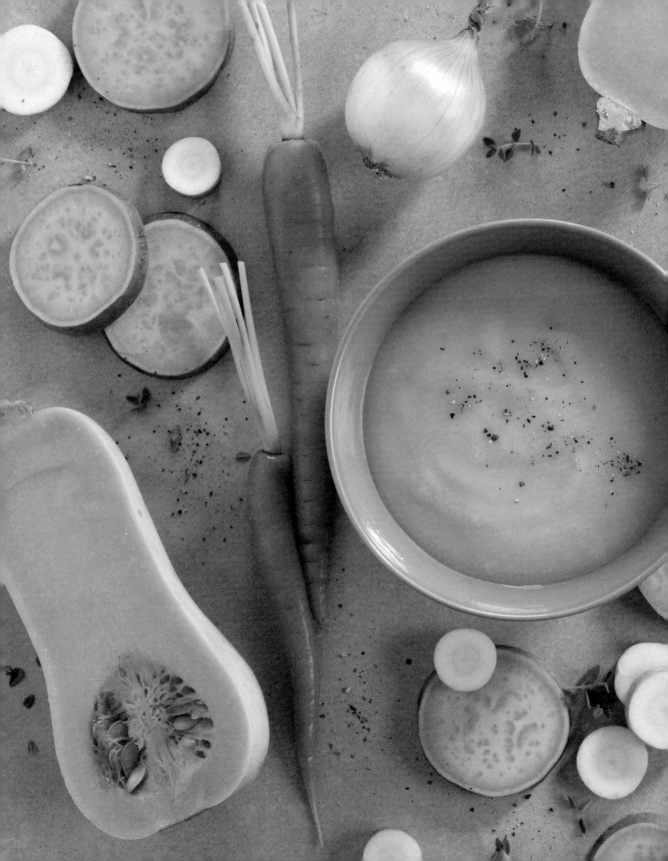

WINTER ROOT VEGETABLE SOUP

This **smooth and creamy** combination highlights **hearty, vitamin-rich root vegetables** accented with **fresh thyme**. Warm and satisfying, it's delicious on a cold winter night. Serve hot.

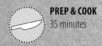 **PREP & COOK**
35 minutes

 QUANTITY
Makes 10 cups
Serving size 2 cups

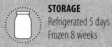 **STORAGE**
Refrigerated 5 days
Frozen 8 weeks

INGREDIENTS

3 TB. coconut oil
3 cups onion, diced
2 TB. garlic, minced
1 cup sweet potato, peeled and diced
1 cup butternut squash, peeled and diced
1 cup carrot, peeled and diced
1⅓ cups parsnip, peeled and diced
1 cup celeriac, peeled and diced
8 cups purified water
1 tsp. fresh thyme, minced
1 tsp. salt
½ tsp. pepper

METHOD

1 In a large stockpot, heat coconut oil over medium heat for 2 minutes. Add onion and garlic and cook until onion is translucent, about 5 minutes.

2 Add sweet potato, butternut squash, carrot, parsnip, celeriac, and water. Increase heat and bring to a boil, then reduce heat and simmer for 10 minutes or until vegetables are cooked through. Remove from heat.

3 Transfer contents of pot to blender and add thyme. Carefully purée until smooth and well combined. Season with salt and pepper.

NUTRITION PER SERVING

calories	178
total fat	4g
cholesterol	0mg
sodium	538mg
carbohydrate	36g
dietary fiber	8g
sugars	12g
protein	4g

DETOXIFY
5-DAY CLEANSE

It's difficult to control your exposure to harmful environmental toxins, but you can work to combat them through dietary changes. These soups contain ingredients with detoxifying properties that work to cleanse the liver, purify the blood, and neutralize damaging compounds.

Follow for 5 days for optimal results. Incorporate a 1-day cleanse on a weekly basis for maintenance.

Shopping List

Fridge/Freezer
Beets (6 medium)
Onions (12)
Red onion (1)
Carrots (11 medium)
Celery (16 stalks)
Garlic (23 cloves)
Baby spinach (24 cups)
Kale (6 cups, chopped)
Fennel (4 large bulbs)
Zucchini (6 medium)
Broccoli, florets (12 cups)
Arugula (6 cups)
Parsnips (5 medium)
Fresh ginger (1 [3-in.; 7.5cm] piece)
Granny Smith apples (6 large)
Lemons (4)
Orange juice, fresh squeezed (3 cups)
Fresh basil (1½ cups, chopped)
Fresh mint (1½ cups, chopped)

Pantry
Olive oil (3 TB.)
Coconut oil (1 cup + 1 TB.)
Artichoke hearts (3 [14-oz.; 400g] cans)
Purified water (14 qt.; 14l)
Vanilla extract (1½ TB.)
Cinnamon sticks (2)
Red pepper flakes (1½ tsp.)
Salt
Pepper

PREPARATION			DURING THE CLEANSE	
1 WEEK BEFORE	**2 DAYS BEFORE**	**1 DAY BEFORE**	**DAILY SOUPS**	**CLEANSE BOOSTERS**
★ Make **Broccoli Arugula Soup** (triple batch); freeze in 2-cup portions. RECIPE PAGE 143	★ Make **Fennel & Zucchini Soup** (triple batch); refrigerate in 2-cup portions. RECIPE PAGE 129	★ Make **Beet, Orange, & Basil Soup** (triple batch); refrigerate in 2-cup portions. RECIPE PAGE 40	**BREAKFAST** Beet, Orange, & Basil Soup (2 cups)	★ Drink 2 cups of alkalized water between meals.
★ Make **Artichoke Basil Soup** (triple batch); freeze in 2-cup portions. RECIPE PAGE 75	★ Make **Leafy Greens Detox Soup** (triple batch); refrigerate in 2-cup portions. RECIPE PAGE 116	★ Make **Apple & Parsnip Soup** (double batch); refrigerate in 1-cup portions. RECIPE PAGE 106	**SNACK** Broccoli Arugula Soup (2 cups) **LUNCH** Fennel & Zucchini Soup (2 cups)	★ Perform 30 to 60 minutes of light to moderate exercise daily during cleanse, particularly hot yoga or cardio, to aid in detoxification.
★ Eliminate processed foods and sugar from your diet and focus on whole foods.	★ Eliminate poultry, meat, and dairy from your diet. ★ Focus on vegetable-based meals supplemented with fish, grains, and legumes.	★ Transfer Broccoli Arugula Soup and Artichoke Basil Soup from freezer to refrigerator to thaw. ★ Eliminate all animal products from your diet. ★ Eat vegetable-based meals with some legumes, grains, and nuts. ★ Drink at least 8 cups of water.	**SNACK** Leafy Greens Detox Soup (2 cups) **DINNER** Artichoke Basil Soup (2 cups) **DESSERT** Apple & Parsnip Soup (1 cup) **ALTERNATIVES** Strawberry Chia Soup (breakfast) RECIPE PAGE 45 Red Pepper Chickpea Soup (dinner) RECIPE PAGE 138	★ Receive a colonic treatment halfway through or at the end of your cleanse.

ANCIENT GRAINS SOUP

The **ancient grains** amaranth, freekeh, and quinoa bring a **robust texture** and **earthy flavor** to this rich tomato soup. With a **savory mix** of vegetables, it's **nutritious and satisfying.** Serve hot.

 PREP & COOK
45 minutes

 QUANTITY
Makes 4 cups
Serving size 2 cups

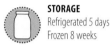 **STORAGE**
Refrigerated 5 days
Frozen 8 weeks

INGREDIENTS

¾ TB. olive oil

½ cup onion, diced

½ cup celery, diced

½ cup carrot, peeled and diced

2 tsp. garlic, minced (about 2 cloves)

1 (14.5-oz; 411g) can diced tomatoes

¼ cup amaranth, cooked

¼ cup freekeh, cooked

¼ cup quinoa, cooked

1¾ cups purified water

1 tsp. parsley, chopped

¼ tsp. salt

¼ tsp. pepper

METHOD

1 In a medium stockpot, heat olive oil over medium heat for 2 minutes. Add onion, celery, carrot, and garlic, and cook until onion is translucent, about 5 minutes.

2 Add tomatoes (with juices), amaranth, freekeh, quinoa, and water. Increase heat and bring to a boil, and then reduce heat and simmer for 15 minutes. Remove from heat.

3 Transfer contents of pot to blender and add parsley. Purée until well combined. Season with salt and pepper.

NUTRITION PER SERVING

calories	220
total fat	7g
cholesterol	0mg
sodium	692mg
carbohydrate	34g
dietary fiber	6g
sugars	9g
protein	6g

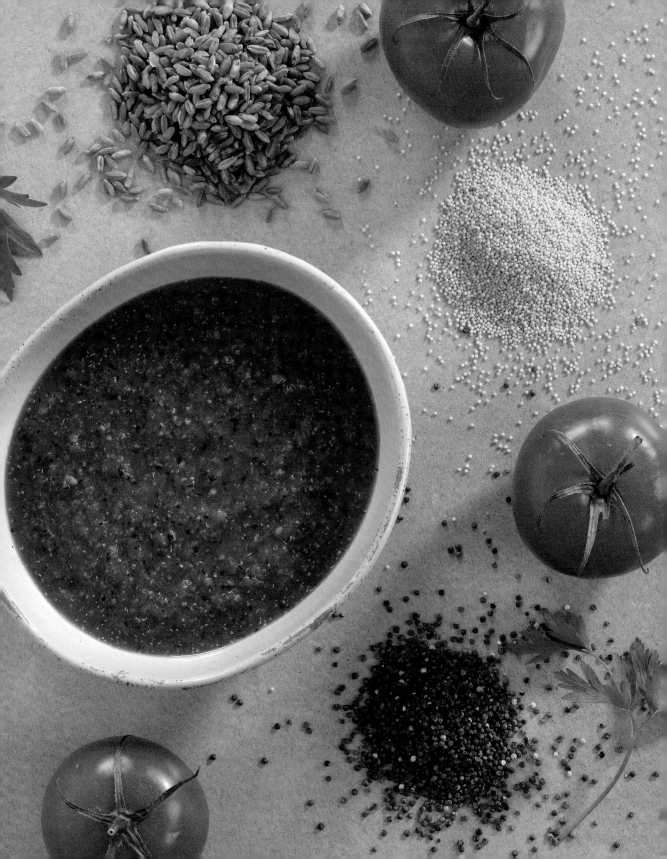

ROASTED SUNCHOKE SOUP

Sunchokes, also called **Jerusalem artichokes,** are a small tuber with a **delicate, slightly sweet flavor.** Roasted alongside **cauliflower,** they yield an **earthy, nutty soup** with a velvety texture. Serve hot.

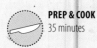 **PREP & COOK**
35 minutes

 QUANTITY
Makes 6 cups
Serving size 2 cups

STORAGE
Refrigerated 5 days
Frozen 8 weeks

INGREDIENTS

2 cups cauliflower florets

1½ cups onion, diced

¼ cup celery, diced

2 cups sunchokes, sliced
  (about 6 sunchokes)

2 TB. olive oil

Juice of ½ lemon

5 cups purified water

3 TB. parsley, minced

¼ tsp. cayenne

½ tsp. salt

¼ tsp. pepper

METHOD

1 Preheat oven to 450°F (230°C). Line a baking sheet with foil.

2 In a medium bowl, combine cauliflower, onion, celery, and sunchokes. Drizzle with olive oil and toss to coat. Spread vegetables on prepared baking sheet and bake for 20 minutes or until they begin to brown.

3 In a blender, combine roasted vegetables, lemon juice, water, parsley, and cayenne. Blend until smooth, adding water if needed to thin. Season with salt and pepper and blend briefly to combine.

NUTRITION PER SERVING

calories	209
total fat	9g
cholesterol	0mg
sodium	423mg
carbohydrate	13g
dietary fiber	5g
sugars	15g
protein	4g

Try using...
2 cups parsnips (peeled and diced) instead of sunchokes, if sunchokes are unavailable.

SPICED CHICKPEA SOUP

This soup features the **spicy, exotic flavors** of cinnamon, cumin, and paprika, along with **hearty chickpeas**. With plenty of protein, it's a **warm and satisfying** meal. Serve hot.

PREP & COOK
35 minutes

QUANTITY
Makes 4 cups
Serving size 2 cups

STORAGE
Refrigerated 5 days
Frozen 8 weeks

INGREDIENTS

- 1½ TB. olive oil
- 1 cup onion, diced
- 1 TB. garlic, minced (about 3 cloves)
- 1 tsp. cumin
- 2 tsp. cinnamon
- ¼ tsp. cayenne
- ½ tsp. paprika
- 1 cup canned diced tomato
- 1 (15-oz.; 425g) can chickpeas, drained and rinsed
- 4 cups purified water
- 1 cup baby spinach
- 1 TB. cilantro, chopped
- ¼ tsp. salt

METHOD

1. In a medium stockpot, heat olive oil over medium heat for 2 minutes. Add onion and garlic and cook until onion is translucent, about 5 minutes. Add cumin, cinnamon, cayenne, paprika, and tomatoes and cook for another 3 minutes.

2. Add chickpeas and water. Increase heat and bring to a boil, then reduce heat, cover, and simmer for 15 minutes. Remove from heat.

3. Transfer contents of pot to blender. Add spinach and cilantro to blender and blend until well combined. Add water to thin if needed. Season with salt and blend briefly to combine.

NUTRITION PER SERVING

calories	296	carbohydrate	54g
total fat	6g	dietary fiber	17g
cholesterol	0mg	sugars	14g
sodium	565mg	protein	13g

RED PEPPER CHICKPEA SOUP

This **vibrant soup** brings together the flavors of **roasted red bell peppers** and **nutty chickpeas** in one creamy, satisfying bowl. Fire-roasted tomatoes add a **savory, slightly smokey** note. Serve hot.

PREP & COOK
30 minutes

QUANTITY
Makes 4 cups
Serving size 2 cups

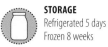
STORAGE
Refrigerated 5 days
Frozen 8 weeks

INGREDIENTS

1½ TB. olive oil

1½ cups onion, diced

2 TB. garlic, minced (about 2 cloves)

½ cup canned fire-roasted diced tomatoes

1½ cups roasted red pepper, rinsed and drained

½ cup canned chickpeas, rinsed and drained

4 cups purified water

2 TB. parsley, minced

¼ tsp. salt

METHOD

1 In a medium stockpot, heat olive oil over medium heat for 2 minutes. Add onion and garlic and cook until onion is translucent, about 5 minutes.

2 Add diced tomatoes, roasted red pepper, chickpeas, and water. Increase heat and bring to a boil, then reduce heat and cover. Simmer for 10 minutes. Remove from heat.

3 Transfer contents of pot to blender and purée until smooth. Add parsley and salt, and blend briefly to combine.

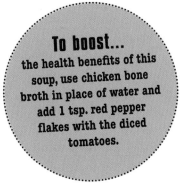

To boost... the health benefits of this soup, use chicken bone broth in place of water and add 1 tsp. red pepper flakes with the diced tomatoes.

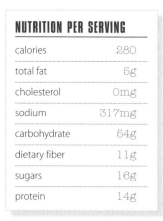

NUTRITION PER SERVING

calories	280
total fat	5g
cholesterol	0mg
sodium	317mg
carbohydrate	54g
dietary fiber	11g
sugars	16g
protein	14g

Red bell pepper is an excellent source of antioxidants and has more vitamin C per serving than an orange.

CHAI SPICED ALMOND SOUP

With **star anise, cinnamon, ginger,** and **cardamom,** this soup tastes like a spicy, dairy-free version of your **favorite chai latte.** Almonds add a **creamy texture** as well as **nourishing protein.** Serve chilled.

PREP & COOK
12 hours

QUANTITY
Makes 4 cups
Serving size 1 cup

STORAGE
Refrigerated 5 days
Frozen 8 weeks

INGREDIENTS

2 TB. decaffeinated loose-leaf black tea, or 2 decaffeinated black tea bags

4 cups purified water

1 cup raw almonds

2 cinnamon sticks

1 star anise

4 TB. agave nectar

2 tsp. vanilla, or seeds from 1 vanilla bean

1½ TB. fresh ginger, grated

¾ tsp. ground cardamom

½ tsp. cracked black pepper

½ tsp. cinnamon

METHOD

1 Place tea in a 1-quart (1l) heat-resistant jar. In a saucepan or kettle, bring water to boil over high heat. Pour boiling water over tea. Steep for 4 to 5 minutes. Strain and discard tea leaves.

2 Add almonds, cinnamon sticks, and star anise to tea. Cool and refrigerate overnight.

3 Remove cinnamon sticks and star anise from tea. Transfer contents of jar to blender and add agave nectar, vanilla, ginger, cardamom, black pepper, and cinnamon. Blend until smooth.

NUTRITION PER SERVING	
calories	287
total fat	18g
cholesterol	0mg
sodium	6mg
carbohydrate	26g
dietary fiber	5g
sugars	16g
protein	8g

For a sweet,...
earthy flavor, try rooibos tea instead of black tea.

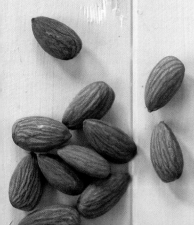

MUSHROOM & MILLET SOUP

This soup features the **ancient grain millet,** which is rich in fiber and protein as well as vitamin B3. Paired with **savory, earthy mushrooms,** it makes for a **satisfying yet low-calorie** meal. Serve hot.

PREP & COOK
35 minutes

QUANTITY
Makes 4 cups
Serving size 2 cups

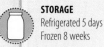

STORAGE
Refrigerated 5 days
Frozen 8 weeks

INGREDIENTS

1 TB. olive oil
1 cup onion, diced
1 TB. garlic, minced
  (about 3 cloves)
4 cups cremini mushrooms,
  diced
3 cups purified water
¼ cup millet, cooked
Juice of ½ lemon
2 TB. parsley, minced
½ tsp. fresh thyme, minced
¾ tsp. salt
¼ tsp. pepper
½ tsp. truffle oil (optional)

METHOD

1 In a medium stockpot, heat olive oil over medium heat for 2 minutes. Add onion and garlic and cook until onion is translucent, about 5 minutes.

2 Add mushrooms and water. Increase heat and bring to boil, then reduce heat and simmer for 10 minutes or until mushrooms are cooked through. Remove from heat.

3 Transfer contents of pot to blender, and add millet, lemon juice, parsley, and thyme. Purée until smooth. Season with salt and pepper, and add truffle oil, if using. Blend briefly to combine.

NUTRITION PER SERVING

calories	115	carbohydrate	22g
total fat	2g	dietary fiber	3g
cholesterol	0mg	sugars	7g
sodium	885mg	protein	6g

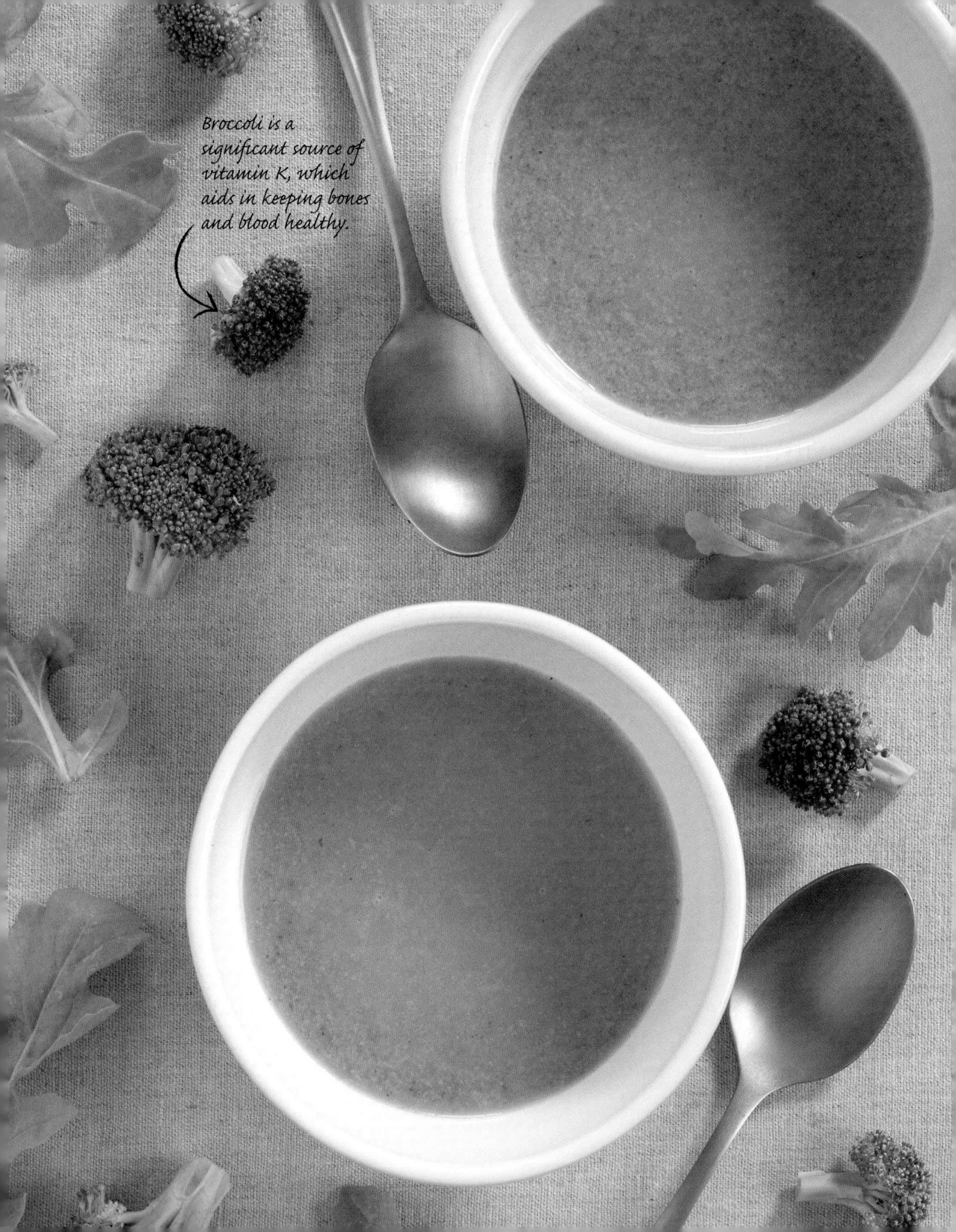

Broccoli is a
significant source of
vitamin K, which
aids in keeping bones
and blood healthy.

BROCCOLI ARUGULA SOUP

Hearty broccoli and **peppery arugula** come together in this **light-bodied soup** that is both **energizing and detoxifying.** A squeeze of lemon adds **brightness and zest.** Serve hot.

 PREP & COOK
20 minutes

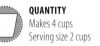 **QUANTITY**
Makes 4 cups
Serving size 2 cups

 STORAGE
Refrigerated 5 days
Frozen 8 weeks

INGREDIENTS

1 TB. coconut oil

2 tsp. garlic, minced (about 2 cloves)

1 cup onion, diced

4 cups broccoli florets

3¾ cups purified water

2 cups baby arugula, tightly packed

¼ tsp. salt

⅛ tsp. pepper

1 wedge lemon

METHOD

1 In a medium stockpot, heat coconut oil over medium heat for 2 minutes. Add onion and garlic, and cook until onion is translucent, about 5 minutes.

2 Add broccoli and water to pot. Increase heat and bring to a boil, then reduce heat, cover, and simmer for 5 minutes or until broccoli is cooked through. Remove from heat.

3 Transfer contents of pot to blender and add arugula. Blend until smooth and well combined. Season with salt and pepper and finish with a squeeze of lemon.

NUTRITION PER SERVING

calories	117
total fat	2g
cholesterol	0mg
sodium	69mg
carbohydrate	22g
dietary fiber	7g
sugars	7g
protein	7g

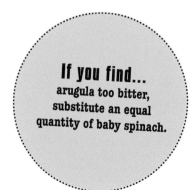

If you find...
arugula too bitter,
substitute an equal
quantity of baby spinach.

IMMUNE BOOST
3-DAY CLEANSE

Your immune system monitors and protects against disease and infection on a daily basis. Poor diet and lifestyle choices can negatively affect your immune system, and a weakened immune system can leave your body susceptible to dysfunctions and more serious infections.

Follow for 3 days to strengthen immunity.

Shopping List

Fridge/Freezer
Onions (6)
Celery (4 stalks)
Carrots (11 medium)
Garlic (19 cloves)
Fennel (3 bulbs)
Strawberries (6 cups)
Bananas (4)
Parsley (1 bunch)
Fresh dill (3 TB., minced)
Ginger (½ tsp., grated)
Bone-in chicken parts (2 lb.; 1kg)
Chicken feet (2 lb.; 1kg)

Pantry
Olive oil (9 TB.)
Coconut oil (1½ TB.)
Apple cider vinegar (2 TB.)
Red wine vinegar (4 tsp.)
Purified water (9 qt.; 9l)
Coconut water (4 cups)
Light coconut milk (½ cup)
Fire-roasted diced tomatoes (1 [14.5-oz.; 411g] can)
Diced tomatoes (2 [14.5-oz.; 411g] cans)
Roasted red peppers (6 cups)
Flax seed, ground (4 tsp.)
Chia seeds (4 tsp.)
Walnuts (2 cups)
Almonds, blanched (1 cup)
Agave nectar (3 tsp.)
Bay leaf (1)
Red pepper flakes (½ tsp.)
Cayenne (1 tsp.)
Curry powder (2 TB.)
Cinnamon sticks (2)
Salt
pepper

PREPARATION			DURING THE CLEANSE	
1 WEEK BEFORE	**2 DAYS BEFORE**	**1 DAY BEFORE**	**DAILY SOUPS**	**CLEANSE BOOSTERS**
★ Make **Jalapeño Chicken Broth** (single batch); freeze in 2-cup portions. RECIPE PAGE 156	★ Make **Curried Carrot Soup** (double batch); refrigerate in 2-cup portions. RECIPE PAGE 38	★ Make **Strawberry Chia Soup** (double batch); refrigerate in 2-cup portions. RECIPE PAGE 45	**BREAKFAST** Strawberry Chia Soup (2 cups)	★ Drink 2 cups of alkalized water between meals
★ Make **Red Pepper Romesco Soup** (double batch); freeze in 2-cup portions. RECIPE PAGE 63	★ Make **Tomato Broth with Dill** (single batch); refrigerate in 2-cup portions. RECIPE PAGE 173	★ **Banana Walnut Soup** (double batch); refrigerate in 1-cup portions. RECIPE PAGE 107	**SNACK** Jalapeño Chicken Broth (2 cups)	★ Perform 30 to 60 minutes of light to moderate exercise daily during cleanse.
★ Eliminate processed foods and sugar from your diet and focus on whole foods.	★ Eliminate poultry, meat, and dairy from your diet.	★ Transfer Jalapeño Chicken Broth and Red Pepper Romesco Soup from freezer to refrigerator to thaw.	**LUNCH** Red Pepper Romesco Soup (2 cups)	
	★ Focus on vegetable-based meals supplemented with fish, grains, and legumes.	★ Eat vegetable-based meals with some legumes, grains, and nuts.	**SNACK** Curried Carrot Soup (2 cups)	
			DINNER Tomato Broth with Dill (2 cups)	
		★ Drink at least 8 cups of water.	**DESSERT** Banana Walnut Soup (1 cup)	
			ALTERNATIVES Citrus Soup with Lavender (breakfast) RECIPE PAGE 150	
			Asparagus Soup with Mint (lunch) RECIPE PAGE 51	

CARROT & FENNEL SOUP

Roasting with **a touch of honey** brings out the **earthy sweetness** of **carrots and fennel,** which is complemented by savory **fresh thyme** in this **creamy, comforting soup.** Serve hot.

 PREP & COOK
30 minutes

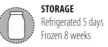 **QUANTITY**
Makes 4 cups
Serving size 2 cups

STORAGE
Refrigerated 5 days
Frozen 8 weeks

INGREDIENTS

2 cups carrot, peeled
   and diced

2 cups fennel, diced

1 cup onion, diced

2 TB. coconut oil

2 TB. honey

4 cups purified water

½ tsp. fresh thyme,
   minced

¼ tsp. salt

¼ tsp. pepper

METHOD

1 Preheat oven to 425°F (220°C). Line a baking sheet with foil.

2 In a medium bowl, combine carrot, fennel, and onion. Drizzle with coconut oil and honey and toss to combine. Spread vegetables on prepared baking sheet and roast for 12 to 15 minutes or until they begin to caramelize.

3 In a blender, combine roasted vegetables, water, and thyme. Blend until smooth. Season with salt and pepper and heat before serving if needed.

NUTRITION PER SERVING

calories	293
total fat	14g
cholesterol	0mg
sodium	428mg
carbohydrate	43g
dietary fiber	8g
sugars	13g
protein	3g

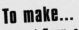
To make...
Zesty Carrot Soup, add ½ cup Greek yogurt to blender, replace thyme with 2 TB. minced cilantro, add ½ tsp. cumin, and finish with a squirt of lime juice.

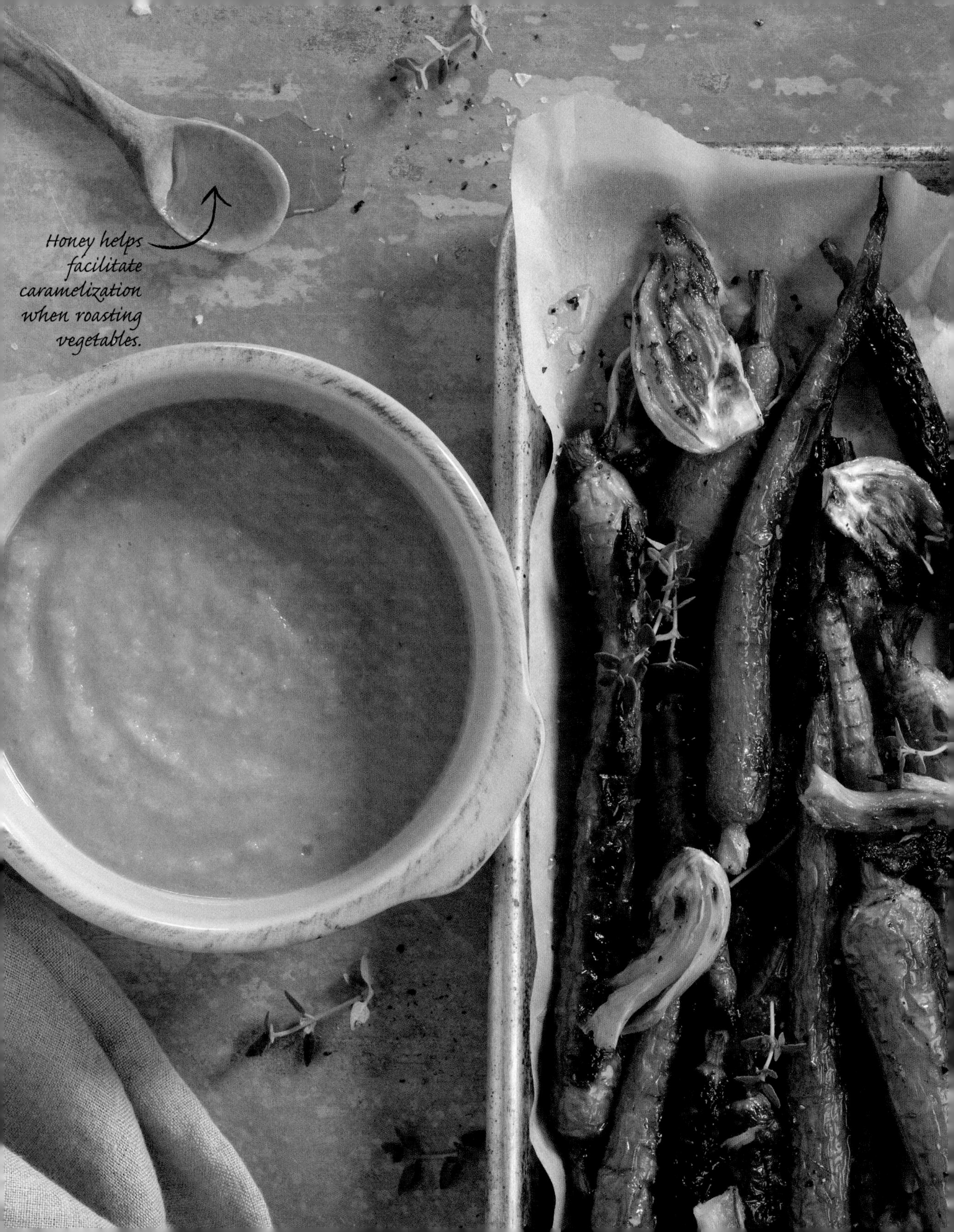

Honey helps
facilitate
caramelization
when roasting
vegetables.

BUTTERNUT BLACK BEAN SOUP

Chunks of **sweet butternut squash** are complemented by a **smokey tomato broth** and **robust black beans** in this fiber-rich, filling soup. Chile powder adds a hint of **warming spice.** Serve hot.

PREP & COOK
45 minutes

QUANTITY
Makes 4 cups
Serving size 2 cups

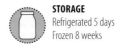

STORAGE
Refrigerated 5 days
Frozen 8 weeks

INGREDIENTS

2 TB. olive oil

¾ cup onion, diced

2½ TB. garlic, minced
(about 7 cloves)

1½ tsp. tomato paste

½ cup canned fire-roasted
diced tomatoes

2½ cups purified water

1½ tsp. chili powder

¾ tsp. coriander

¾ tsp. cumin

1 tsp. chile de árbol
(optional)

1 cup butternut squash,
peeled and cubed

1 cup canned black beans,
drained and rinsed

1½ TB. cilantro, minced

Juice of 1 lime

¼ tsp. salt

METHOD

1 In a medium stockpot, heat olive oil over medium heat for 2 minutes. Add onion and garlic, and cook until onion is translucent, about 5 minutes. Stir in tomato paste and cook for another 3 minutes.

2 Add diced tomatoes, water, chili powder, coriander, cumin, chile de árbol (if using), butternut squash, and black beans.

3 Increase heat and bring to a boil, then reduce heat, cover, and simmer until butternut squash is cooked through, about 20 minutes.

4 Before serving, stir in cilantro and lime juice. Season with salt to taste.

NUTRITION PER SERVING	
calories	232
total fat	4g
cholesterol	0mg
sodium	534mg
carbohydrate	43g
dietary fiber	13g
sugars	6g
protein	11g

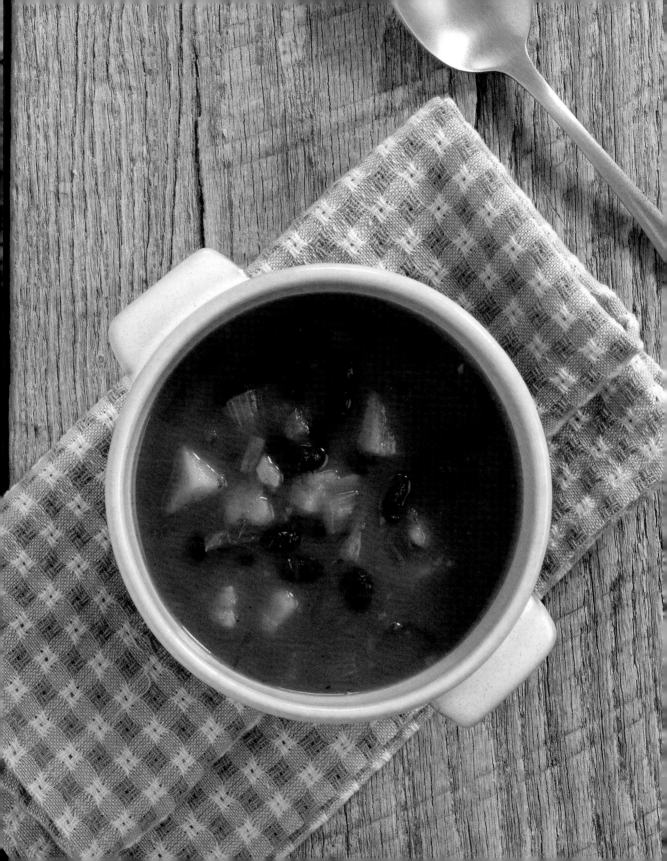

CITRUS SOUP WITH LAVENDER

Bright citrus flavors of orange and grapefruit are combined with nutty chia and **soothing lavender** to create this **fresh, invigorating soup.** Enjoy for breakfast or dessert. Serve chilled.

 PREP & COOK
20 minutes

 QUANTITY
Makes 3 cups
Serving size 1 cup

STORAGE
Refrigerated 5 days
Frozen 8 weeks

INGREDIENTS

3 oranges

2 grapefruits

⅔ cup coconut water

2 tsp. fresh lavender, minced

2 TB. chia seeds

METHOD

1 Supreme oranges and grapefruits by carefully slicing away the rinds and removing the membranes. Reserve the juice.

2 In a blender, combine orange supremes, grapefruit supremes, reserved citrus juice, coconut water, and lavender. Purée until smooth, about 30 seconds.

3 If desired, transfer blending vessel to refrigerator to chill for 30 minutes. Before serving, stir in chia seeds and let sit until chia seeds are plump, about 10 minutes.

NUTRITION PER SERVING

calories	185
total fat	3g
cholesterol	0mg
sodium	15mg
carbohydrate	39g
dietary fiber	8g
sugars	25g
protein	4g

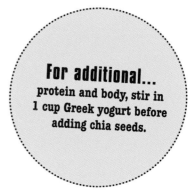

For additional... protein and body, stir in 1 cup Greek yogurt before adding chia seeds.

Lavender has natural anti-inflammatory benefits and aids in digestion.

Flavonoids in citrus fruits can neutralize free radicals.

NUTMEG SWEET POTATO SOUP

This **cozy soup** tastes like the holidays, with the **warm spice of nutmeg**, hearty **sweet potatoes**, and a **touch of maple syrup**. Smooth and **creamy**, it's a delicious and healthy treat. Serve hot.

PREP & COOK
45 minutes

QUANTITY
Makes 4 cups
Serving size 2 cups

STORAGE
Refrigerated 5 days
Frozen 8 weeks

INGREDIENTS

1½ TB. coconut oil

½ cup celery, diced

1½ cups onion, diced

1 tsp. garlic, minced (about 1 clove)

4 cups purified water

3 cups sweet potato, peeled and cubed

4 TB. pure maple syrup

½ tsp. fresh nutmeg, grated

⅛ tsp. salt

METHOD

1 In a medium stockpot, heat coconut oil over medium heat for 2 minutes. Add celery, onion, and garlic. Cook until onion becomes translucent, about 5 minutes.

2 Add water and sweet potato. Increase heat and bring to a boil, then reduce heat to a simmer and cover. Simmer until sweet potatoes are cooked through, about 15 minutes. Remove from heat.

3 Add contents of pot to blender along with maple syrup and nutmeg. Blend until smooth. Season with salt and blend briefly to combine.

NUTRITION PER SERVING

calories	344
total fat	2g
cholesterol	0mg
sodium	285mg
carbohydrate	80g
dietary fiber	9g
sugars	38g
protein	5g

For a lighter flavor...
use 3 cups butternut squash (peeled and cubed) instead of sweet potatoes.

The natural sugars in sweet potatoes release slowly, ensuring an extended source of energy.

Unlike most other sweeteners, pure maple syrup does not cause spikes in blood sugar.

6
BROTHS & CONSOMMÉS

Digestive health and anti-inflammatory cleanses, which utilize restorative broths and consommés, are featured here. The recipes in this part include both vegetable and protein-based ingredients that are delicious on their own or as a base for other soups.

JALAPEÑO CHICKEN BROTH

Nourishing bone broth is a comforting snack on its own or a nutrient-rich **addition to soups.** This recipe for **basic chicken bone broth** includes the optional addition of **lime and jalapeños.** Serve hot.

 PREP & COOK
7 to 24 hours

 QUANTITY
Makes 6 cups
Serving size 2 cups

 STORAGE
Refrigerated 5 days
Frozen 8 weeks

INGREDIENTS

2 TB. olive oil

2 lb. (1kg) bone-in chicken parts (legs, backs, and necks)

2 lb. (1kg) chicken feet

12 cups purified water

2 TB. apple cider vinegar

1 cup onion, chopped

1 cup celery, chopped

1 cup carrot, chopped

8 cloves garlic, peeled

1 bay leaf

½ bunch parsley

2 TB. jalapeño pepper, thinly sliced (optional)

Juice of 4 limes (optional)

½ tsp. salt

½ tsp. pepper

METHOD

1 In a large stockpot, heat olive oil over medium heat for 2 minutes. Add chicken pieces and cook for 8 minutes, turning to brown on all sides.

2 Add water to cover chicken by 3 to 4 inches (7.5–10cm). Add apple cider vinegar and cook over medium-high heat until boiling, about 35 minutes.

3 Reduce heat to simmer and cover. Simmer for at least 6 hours and up to 24 hours. Skim broth intermittently, and add water as needed to ensure bones remain covered.

4 Two hours before removing broth from the stove, add onion, celery, carrot, garlic, bay leaf, and parsley. Cook for remaining 2 hours, and then remove pot from heat.

5 Strain broth, discarding solids. Add jalapeños and lime juice (if using), and salt and pepper. Transfer to refrigerator to cool. Once cool, skim fat from surface. Heat before serving.

NUTRITION PER SERVING			
calories	68	carbohydrate	15g
total fat	3g	dietary fiber	1g
cholestoral	0mg	sugars	3g
sodium	404mg	protein	1g

The capsaicin in jalapeños is a powerful inflammation-fighting compound.

SESAME VEGETABLE BROTH

The **rich flavor of toasted sesame oil** is perfectly balanced with the bright background **notes of lime** in this Asian-inspired broth. **Ginger provides spice** and **promotes healthy digestion.** Serve hot.

 PREP & COOK
1 hour

 QUANTITY
Makes 6 cups
Serving size 2 cups

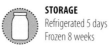 **STORAGE**
Refrigerated 5 days
Frozen 8 weeks

INGREDIENTS

2 TB. olive oil

1 cup onion, chopped

1 cup lemongrass, roughly chopped

1 cup ginger, unpeeled and roughly chopped

1 cup carrot, chopped

5 cloves garlic, whole

8 cups purified water

3 TB. tamari

Juice of 3 limes

1 tsp. toasted sesame oil

½ cup green onion, thinly sliced

METHOD

1 In a medium stockpot, heat olive oil over medium heat for 2 minutes. Add onion, lemongrass, ginger, carrot, and garlic. Cook until onion is translucent, about 5 minutes.

2 Add water, increase heat, and bring to a boil. Reduce heat, cover, and simmer for 40 minutes. Remove from heat.

3 Strain broth and discard vegetables. Add tamari, lime juice, and sesame oil. Top with green onions.

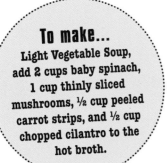

To make...
Light Vegetable Soup,
add 2 cups baby spinach,
1 cup thinly sliced
mushrooms, ½ cup peeled
carrot strips, and ½ cup
chopped cilantro to the
hot broth.

NUTRITION PER SERVING

calories	76
total fat	4g
cholesterol	10mg
sodium	2,854mg
carbohydrate	7g
dietary fiber	0g
sugars	3g
protein	5g

This warming broth
makes an excellent base
for vegetable soups.

Citrusy lemongrass adds a boost of folate, folic acid, and other minerals.

CARROT CONSOMMÉ

The **mild citrus flavor** of lemongrass complements the natural **sweetness of carrots** in this **aromatic consommé.** An excellent source of vitamin C, it's an **immume-boosting** tonic for cold season. Serve hot.

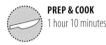
PREP & COOK
1 hour 10 minutes

QUANTITY
Makes 6 cups
Serving size 2 cups

STORAGE
Refrigerated 5 days
Frozen 8 weeks

INGREDIENTS

5 egg whites

3 cups carrot, peeled and grated

¾ cup lemongrass, thinly sliced

½ cup ginger, chopped

8 cups fresh carrot juice, chilled

2 TB. cilantro, minced

1 tsp. lime zest

½ tsp. salt

METHOD

1 In a small bowl, lightly beat egg whites. Add beaten egg whites to a medium stockpot along with grated carrots, lemongrass, ginger, and carrot juice. Stir to combine.

2 Bring the mixture to a simmer over medium heat, stirring frequently. Within about 20 minutes a "raft" should form at the top. With a spoon, gently break a hole in the middle to allow the consommé to simmer.

3 Reduce heat to medium-low and continue to simmer for 30 minutes. Remove from heat.

4 Line a mesh sieve with cheesecloth or a coffee filter, and place over a large bowl or pot. Gently ladle the consommé into strainer to remove vegetable solids.

5 Add cilantro, lime zest, and salt to strained consommé. Warm before serving, if needed.

NUTRITION PER SERVING

calories	361
total fat	2g
cholesterol	0mg
sodium	983mg
carbohydrate	78g
dietary fiber	9g
sugars	31g
protein	14g

SHIITAKE GINGER BROTH

This **umami-rich broth** is earthy and satisfying. Shiitakes provide B-complex vitamins along with a **variety of minerals**. Ginger aids in digestion and has **anti-inflammatory benefits**. Serve hot.

 PREP & COOK
45 minutes

 QUANTITY
Makes 6 cups
Serving size 2 cups

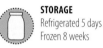 **STORAGE**
Refrigerated 5 days
Frozen 8 weeks

INGREDIENTS

1 TB. olive oil

1 cup onion, chopped

½ cup carrot, peeled and chopped

1 cup fresh ginger, roughly chopped

1 (1-in.; 2.5cm) piece fresh ginger, grated

5 cloves garlic, whole

2 cups shiitake mushrooms, quartered

5 stems parsley

8 cups purified water

¼ cup tamari

METHOD

1 In a medium stockpot, heat olive oil over medium heat for 2 minutes. Add onion, carrot, 1 cup chopped ginger, and garlic. Cook until onion is translucent, about 5 minutes.

2 Add shiitake mushrooms, parsley, and water to pot. Increase heat and bring to boil, and then reduce heat, cover, and simmer for 30 minutes. Remove from heat.

3 Line a mesh sieve with cheesecloth and strain broth, discarding vegetable solids. Stir in tamari and fresh grated ginger. Heat before serving if needed.

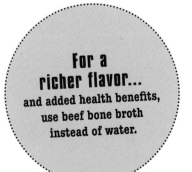

For a richer flavor... and added health benefits, use beef bone broth instead of water.

NUTRITION PER SERVING	
calories	144
total fat	2g
cholesterol	0mg
sodium	1,318mg
carbohydrate	30g
dietary fiber	5g
sugars	8g
protein	6g

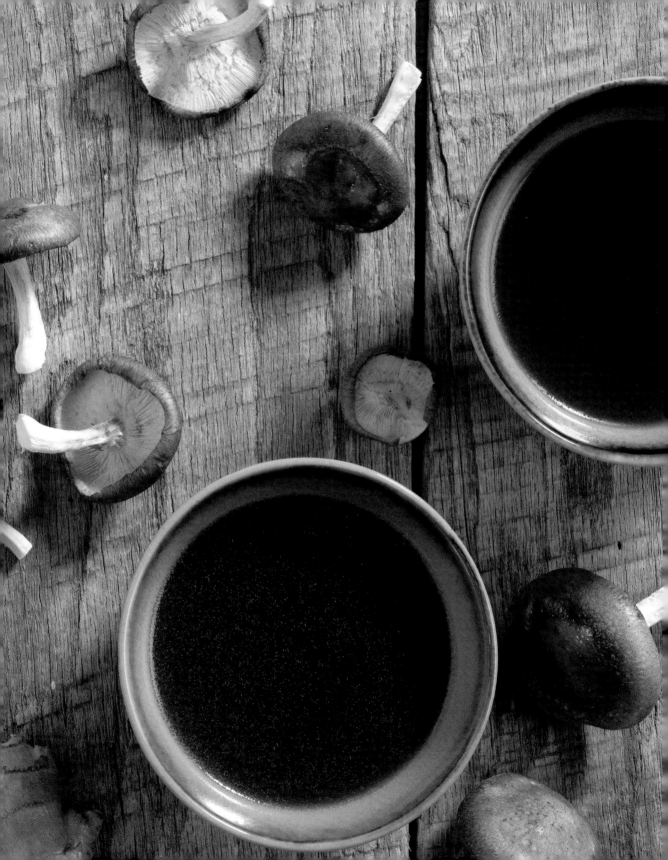

DIGESTIVE HEALTH
5-DAY CLEANSE

Flatten your belly, ease pain and bloating, and aid digestion with this restorative cleanse. Processed foods, fried foods, acidic foods, and dairy can all contribute to digestive issues. This cleanse focuses on hydrating veggies and fiber-rich foods that work to cleanse, hydrate, and restore the digestive system.

Follow for 5 days.

Shopping List

Fridge/Freezer
Leeks (2 cups, diced)
Carrots (4 medium)
Celery (6 stalks)
Garlic (33 cloves)
Onions (6)
Fennel (7 bulbs)
Zucchini (3)
Butternut squash (1 medium)
Baby spinach (9 cups)
Raspberries (3 cups)
Lemon (1)
Limes (6)
Grapefruits (9)
Papaya (9 cups, cubed)
Cilantro (1 bunch)
Vanilla yogurt (1 cup)

Pantry
Olive oil (½ cup)
Coconut oil (3 TB.)
French green lentils (2 cups)
Unsweetened coconut flakes (3 cups)
Purified water (10 qt.; 10l)
Coconut water (7½ cups)
Hemp seeds (8 TB.)
Tomato paste (4½ tsp.)
Fire-roasted diced tomatoes (1 [14.5-oz.; 411g] can)
Black beans (2 [15-oz.; 425g] cans)
Agave nectar (2 TB.)
Spirulina powder (4½ tsp.)
Chili powder (4½ tsp.)
Ground coriander (2¼ tsp.)
Ground cumin (2¼ tsp.)
Salt
Pepper

PREPARATION			DURING THE CLEANSE	
1 WEEK BEFORE	**2 DAYS BEFORE**	**1 DAY BEFORE**	**DAILY SOUPS**	**CLEANSE BOOSTERS**
★ Make **French Lentil Soup** (double batch); freeze in 2-cup portions. RECIPE PAGE 113	★ Make **Fennel & Zucchini Soup** (triple batch); refrigerate in 2-cup portions. RECIPE PAGE 129	★ Make **Papaya & Spinach Soup** (triple batch); refrigerate in 2-cup portions. RECIPE PAGE 71	**BREAKFAST** Papaya & Spinach Soup (2 cups)	★ Drink 2 cups of alkalized water between meals.
★ Make **Butternut Black Bean Soup** (triple batch); freeze in 2-cup portions. RECIPE PAGE 148	★ Make **Grapefruit & Fennel Soup** (triple batch); refrigerate in 2-cup portions. RECIPE PAGE 114	★ Make **Raspberry Coconut Soup** (double batch); refrigerate in 1-cup portions. RECIPE PAGE 87	**SNACK** Fennel & Zucchini Soup (2 cups) **LUNCH** French Lentil Soup (2 cups)	★ Perform 30 to 60 minutes of light to moderate exercise daily during cleanse. Yoga in particular is very good for improving digestion.
★ Eliminate processed foods and sugar from your diet and focus on whole foods.	★ Eliminate poultry, meat, and dairy from your diet.	★ Transfer French Lentil Soup and Butternut Black Bean Soup from freezer to refrigerator to thaw.	**SNACK** Grapefruit & Fennel Soup (2 cups) **DINNER** Butternut Black Bean Soup (2 cups)	★ Receive a colonic treatment halfway through or at the end of your cleanse.
	★ Focus on vegetable-based meals supplemented with fish, grains, and legumes.	★ Eliminate all animal products from your diet.	**DESSERT** Raspberry Coconut Soup (1 cup)	
		★ Eat vegetable-based meals with some legumes, grains, and nuts.	**ALTERNATIVES** Mushroom & Millet Soup (dinner) RECIPE PAGE 141	
		★ Drink at least 8 cups of water.	Beet, Orange, & Basil Soup (snack) RECIPE PAGE 40	

GINGER BEEF BONE BROTH

The longer you simmer this **rich, savory** broth, the more **nutrients and minerals** are extracted from the bones. **Ginger** adds a spicy note, but it can be omited to make a **basic beef bone broth.** Serve hot.

PREP & COOK
10 to 48 hours

QUANTITY
Makes 8 cups
Serving size 2 cups

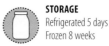

STORAGE
Refrigerated 5 days
Frozen 8 weeks

INGREDIENTS

4 lb. (2kg) beef bones (neck, knucklebones, ribs, shank)

4 TB. olive oil

12 cups purified water

2 TB. apple cider vinegar

1 cup onion, diced

1 cup carrot, diced

1 cup celery, diced with leaves removed

8 cloves garlic, peeled

1 bay leaf

3 TB. tomato paste

½ bunch parsley

4 TB. fresh ginger, grated (optional)

NUTRITION PER SERVING

calories	64
total fat	0g
cholesterol	0mg
sodium	65mg
carbohydrate	14g
dietary fiber	3g
sugars	6g
protein	2g

METHOD

1 Preheat oven to 450°F (230°C) and line a baking sheet with foil. In a large bowl, toss beef bones with olive oil to coat. Spread bones on prepared pan and roast for 20 to 30 minutes. (Roasting intensifies the flavor of the broth.)

2 Using tongs, carefully transfer bones to a large stockpot. Add water, ensuring that water covers bones by at least 3 to 4 inches (7.5–10cm). Stir in apple cider vinegar. Cook over medium-high heat until water begins to boil, about 35 minutes.

3 Reduce heat to simmer and cover. Continue to cook for a minimum of 9 hours or up to 48 hours. Intermittently skim broth to remove the impurities that rise to the top, and add water as needed to keep bones covered.

4 Two hours before removing the broth from the stove, add onion, carrot, celery, garlic, bay leaf, tomato paste, and parsley. Continue to simmer for 2 hours, and then remove pot from heat.

5 Strain broth, discarding vegetables and bones. Stir in fresh grated ginger (if using) and transfer to refrigerator to cool. Once cool, skim hardened fat from surface. Heat before serving and season with salt and pepper if needed.

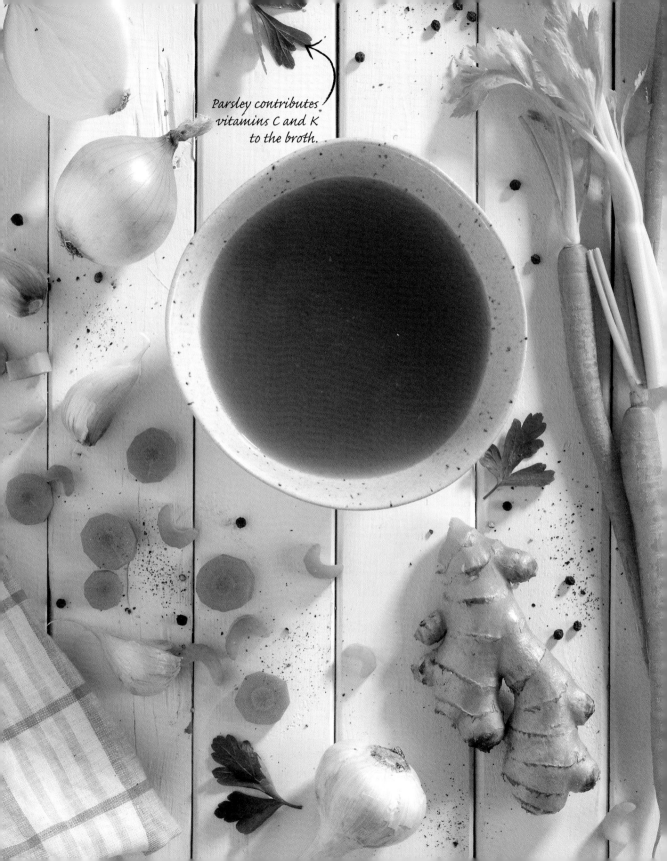

Parsley contributes vitamins C and K to the broth.

ROASTED VEGETABLE STOCK

Roasting vegetables causes them to caramelize, giving this stock **richness** and **depth of flavor.** It makes a **robust vegan base** for soups and stews, or enjoy on its own. Serve hot.

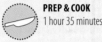 **PREP & COOK**
1 hour 35 minutes

 QUANTITY
Makes 6 cups
Serving size 2 cups

 STORAGE
Refrigerated 5 days
Frozen 8 weeks

INGREDIENTS

¾ cup carrot, chopped

¾ cup leek, chopped

¾ cup celery, chopped

¾ cup portabella mushroom, chopped

8 cloves garlic, peeled

2 TB. olive oil

2 TB. tomato paste

8 cups purified water

5 stems parsley

3 stems thyme

1 tsp. black peppercorns

1 bay leaf

¼ tsp. salt

¼ tsp. pepper

METHOD

1 Preheat oven to 425°F (220°C). In a roasting pan, combine carrots, leeks, celery, and garlic. Drizzle with olive oil and toss to coat. Roast vegetables for 20 minutes or until they begin to brown.

2 Remove vegetables from pan and set aside. Place roasting pan on stovetop across two burners set to medium heat. Add 1 cup water and deglaze pan by running a wooden spoon around the bottom to remove browned vegetables.

3 Transfer liquid to stockpot and add remaining 7 cups water, roasted vegetables, tomato paste, parsley, thyme, peppercorns, and bay leaf. Bring to a boil over high heat and then reduce heat, cover, and simmer for 45 minutes.

4 Strain stock and discard vegetables. Skim off any remaining fat and season with salt and pepper.

NUTRITION PER SERVING

calories	27	carbohydrate	3g
total fat	1g	dietary fiber	1g
cholesterol	0mg	sugars	2g
sodium	203mg	protein	1g

BEEF & POULTRY BONE BROTH

The **mixture of meat bones** brings **layers of flavor,** complexity, and body to this broth. **Rejuvenating and restorative,** it is excellent on its own or as a **base for other soups.** Serve hot.

PREP & COOK
10 to 36 hours

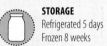

QUANTITY
Makes 8 cups
Serving size 2 cups

STORAGE
Refrigerated 5 days
Frozen 8 weeks

INGREDIENTS

4 TB. olive oil

1½ lb. (680g) beef bones (neck, knucklebones, ribs, shank)

1½ lb. (680g) turkey bones (neck, back)

1½ lb. (680g) chicken bones (neck, back, feet)

12 cups purified water

2 TB. apple cider vinegar

1 cup onion, chopped

1 cup carrot, chopped

1 cup celery, chopped

8 cloves garlic, whole

1 bay leaf

3 TB. tomato paste

½ bunch parsley

½ tsp. salt

¼ tsp. pepper

METHOD

1 Preheat oven to 400°F (200°C). Line a baking sheet with foil. Toss bones with olive oil to coat. Spread bones on prepared pan and roast for 20 to 30 minutes.

2 Using tongs, carefully transfer bones to a large stockpot. Add water, ensuring that water covers bones by at least 3 to 4 inches (7.5–10cm). Stir in apple cider vinegar. Cook over medium-high heat until water boils, about 35 minutes.

3 Reduce heat to simmer and cover. Continue to cook for a minimum of 9 hours or up to 36 hours. Intermittently skim broth, and add water as needed to keep bones covered.

4 Two hours before removing the broth from the stove, add onion, carrot, celery, garlic, bay leaf, tomato paste, and parsley. Continue to simmer for 2 hours.

5 Strain broth, discarding vegetables and bones. Season with salt and pepper to taste.

NUTRITION PER SERVING

calories	14	carbohydrate	3g
total fat	0g	dietary fiber	1g
cholesterol	0mg	sugars	2g
sodium	306mg	protein	1g

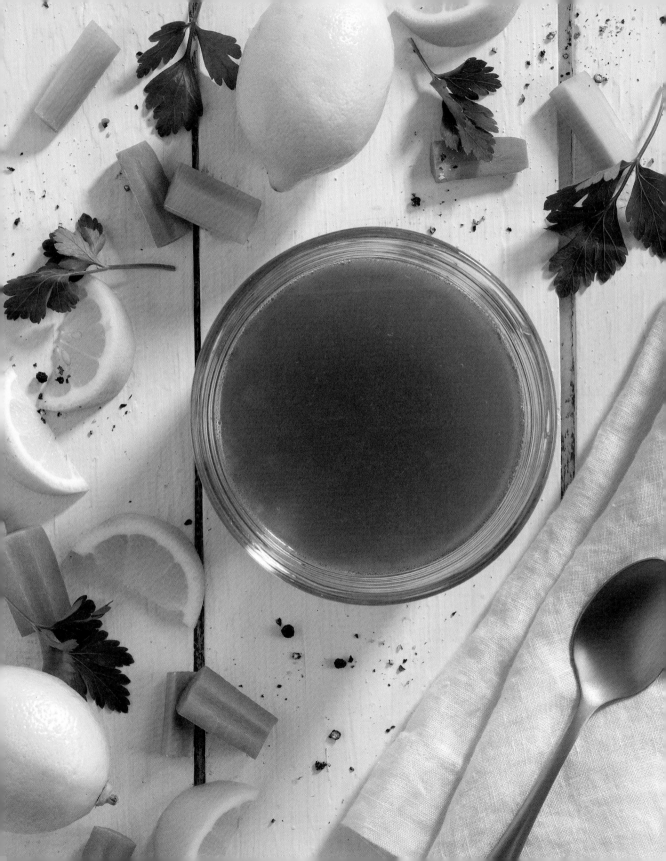

TAMARI & LEMON BROTH

This **light, cleansing broth** is restorative and hydrating. Rich in **vitamins and minerals,** it has **savory depth** from tamari and a **light tanginess** from lemon. Serve hot.

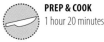 **PREP & COOK**
1 hour 20 minutes

 QUANTITY
Makes 4 cups
Serving size 2 cups

 STORAGE
Refrigerated 5 days
Frozen 8 weeks

INGREDIENTS

1 TB. olive oil

1 cup onion, chopped

1 cup carrot, chopped +
½ cup carrot, sliced into
thin strips

1 cup celery, chopped

3 cloves garlic

¾ cup fresh parsley,
chopped

1 bay leaf

6 cups purified water

½ cup lemon juice (about
5 lemons)

2 TB. tamari

1 cup mushrooms, chopped

1 cup baby spinach

METHOD

1 In a medium stockpot, heat olive oil over medium heat for 2 minutes. Add onion, 1 cup chopped carrot, and celery. Cook until vegetables begin to soften, about 5 minutes.

2 Add water to pot, increase heat, and bring to a boil. Add fresh parsley, garlic, and bay leaf and reduce heat. Cover and simmer for 45 minutes. Remove from heat.

3 Strain broth and discard vegetable solids. Stir in lemon juice, tamari, remaining ½ cup sliced carrots, mushrooms, and spinach. Cover for 10 minutes to allow vegetables to soften in the hot broth.

NUTRITION PER SERVING	
calories	150
total fat	4g
cholesterol	0mg
sodium	1,102mg
carbohydrate	28g
dietary fiber	6g
sugars	10g
protein	6g

TURMERIC CORIANDER BROTH

Homemade bone broth is the basis for this **healing tonic** that features **vibrantly hued turmeric,** which is known for its anti-inflammatory effects and **mood-boosting attributes.** Serve hot.

 PREP & COOK
40 minutes

 QUANTITY
Makes 8 cups
Serving size 2 cups

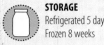 **STORAGE**
Refrigerated 5 days
Frozen 8 weeks

INGREDIENTS

1½ TB. olive oil
½ cup celery, chopped
½ cup carrot, chopped
¾ cup fresh ginger, chopped
8 cloves garlic, peeled
8 cups Beef & Poultry Bone Broth
1 (2-in.; 5cm) piece turmeric, grated
2 TB. tamari
2 tsp. coriander seeds

METHOD

1 In a large stockpot, heat olive oil over medium heat for 2 minutes. Add celery, carrot, ginger, and garlic, and cook for 5 minutes.

2 Add Beef & Poultry Bone Broth (page 169), turmeric, tamari, and coriander to pot. Increase heat and bring to a boil, and then reduce heat, cover, and simmer for 20 minutes. Remove from heat.

3 Using a mesh seive or colander lined with cheesecloth, strain broth, discarding vegetable solids.

NUTRITION PER SERVING

calories	84
total fat	2g
cholesterol	10mg
sodium	618mg
carbohydrate	11g
dietary fiber	2g
sugars	4g
protein	5g

To make...
a vegetarian or vegan version, use Shiitake Ginger Broth instead of bone broth.

TOMATO BROTH WITH DILL

Bright fennel brings out the **natural sweetness of tomatoes** in this delicate broth, while **citrusy dill** adds an aromatic finish. Red pepper flakes provide **mild heat** as well as a **metabolic boost.** Serve hot.

PREP & COOK
1 hour 10 minutes

QUANTITY
Makes 8 cups
Serving size 2 cups

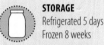

STORAGE
Refrigerated 5 days
Frozen 8 weeks

INGREDIENTS

2 TB. olive oil

⅛ cup onion, diced

⅛ cup celery, diced

⅛ cup carrot, peeled and diced

1 cup fennel, bulb and fronds, diced

1 TB. garlic, minced (about 3 cloves)

1 (14.5-oz.; 411g) can diced fire-roasted tomatoes

½ tsp. red pepper flakes

8 cups purified water

½ tsp. salt

¼ tsp. pepper

3 TB. fresh dill, minced

METHOD

1 In a large stockpot, heat 1 TB. olive oil over medium heat for 2 minutes. Add onion, celery, carrot, fennel, and garlic. Cook until onion is translucent, about 5 minutes. Add tomatoes and red pepper flakes, and cook for 5 minutes.

2 Add water, increase heat, and bring to a boil. Then reduce heat, cover, and simmer for 40 minutes.

3 In batches, transfer contents of pot to a blender and purée until smooth. Strain puréed soup through a fine mesh seive and discard pulp.

4 Season with salt and pepper to taste. Finish with fresh dill and drizzle with remaining 1 TB. olive oil.

NUTRITION PER SERVING

calories	107	carbohydrate	10g
total fat	7g	dietary fiber	3g
cholestoral	0g	sugars	5g
sodium	561g	protein	2g

CHICKEN HERB CONSOMMÉ

Humble chicken soup is elevated with **classic French techniques,** yielding a **delicate consommé** with surprising depth of flavor, finished with a **sprinkling of fresh herbs.** Serve hot.

PREP & COOK
1 hour 40 minutes

QUANTITY
Makes 6 cups
Serving size 2 cups

STORAGE
Refrigerated 5 days
Frozen 8 weeks

INGREDIENTS

2 stems thyme + 1 tsp. thyme, minced

2 stems parsley

1 bay leaf

½ tsp. peppercorns

5 egg whites, chilled

½ cup celery, diced

1 cup carrot, diced

1 cup onion, diced

1 lb. (450g) ground chicken, very chilled

8 cups homemade chicken bone broth, chilled

1 TB. chives, thinly sliced

½ tsp. fresh rosemary

NUTRITION PER SERVING

calories	75
total fat	18g
cholesterol	175mg
sodium	625mg
carbohydrate	13g
dietary fiber	2g
sugars	8g
protein	47g

METHOD

1 Assemble aromatic sachet by placing thyme stems, parsley stems, bay leaf, and peppercorns in a muslin sachet bag.

2 In a small bowl, lightly beat egg whites until slightly frothy.

3 In a large stockpot, combine beaten egg whites, celery, carrot, onion, ground chicken, chicken bone broth (page 156), and aromatic sachet. Bring to a simmer over medium-high heat, stirring occasionally. Within about 25 minutes, a raft of foam should form on the surface.

4 Reduce heat so liquid is barely simmering. With a spoon, gently break a hole in the middle of the raft to allow the consommé to bubble through. Baste the raft with liquid from the center, without breaking it, about every 15 minutes.

5 Simmer until broth is clear and flavor fully develops, about 1 hour. Remove from heat. Line a mesh strainer with cheesecloth or a coffee filter, and place over a large bowl or pot. Carefully ladle broth from hole in raft into strainer.

6 Strained broth should be clear and free of impurities. Top with chives, rosemary, and remaining minced thyme.

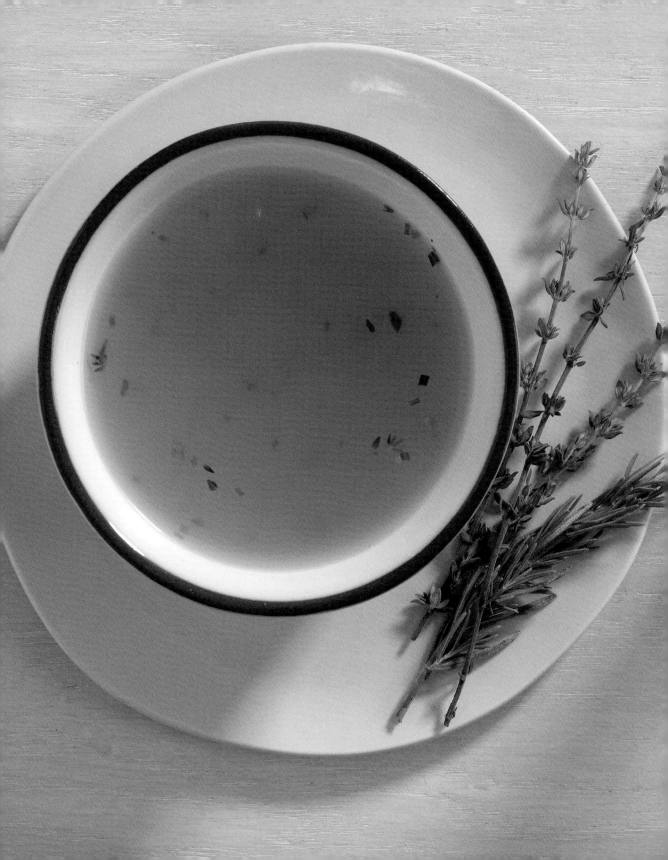

ANTI-INFLAMMATORY
3-DAY CLEANSE

Chronic inflammation has a domino effect that can undermine your overall health. It is directly linked to your diet, and poor choices such as foods high in sugar, saturated fats, trans fats, refined carbohydrates, MSG, and aspartame can cause inflammation to worsen.Use this cleanse to help combat inflammation in the body and for restorative purposes.

Follow for 3 days. Afterward, use as a 1-day cleanse on a weekly basis or incorporate individual soups into your daily diet.

shopping List

Fridge/Freezer
Kale (1 cup, chopped)
Baby spinach (1 cup)
Onions (4)
Red onion (1)
Carrots (7)
Celery (10 stalks)
Red bell pepper (2)
Yellow bell pepper (2)
Orange bell pepper (2)
Cucumber (1)
Beets (3 large)
Garlic (23 cloves)
Fennel (2 bulbs)
Fresh ginger (1 [3-in.; 7.5cm] piece)
Kiwis (4)
Fuji apples (6)
Limes (9)
Green grapes (1 cup, halved)
Mint (6 tsp., minced)
Parsley (1 bunch)
Beef bones (3 lb.; 1.5kg)
Turkey bones (3 lb.; 1.5kg)
Chicken bones (3 lb.; 1.5kg)

Pantry
Olive oil (1 cup)
Apple cider vinegar (4 TB.)
Red wine vinegar (3 TB.)
Purified water (10 qt.; 10l)
Agave nectar (4 tsp.)
Amaranth (1¾ cups, cooked)
Freekeh (¾ cup, cooked)
Quinoa (¾ cup, cooked)
Tomato paste (6 TB.)
Diced tomatoes (6 [14.5-oz.; 411g] cans)
Tomato juice (3 cups)
Coconut water (6½ cups)
Cinnamon sticks (6)
Bay leaves (2)
Salt
Pepper

PREPARATION			**DURING THE CLEANSE**	
1 WEEK BEFORE	**2 DAYS BEFORE**	**1 DAY BEFORE**	**DAILY SOUPS**	**CLEANSE BOOSTERS**
★ Make **Beef & Poultry Bone Broth** (double batch); freeze in 2-cup portions. RECIPE PAGE 169	★ Make **Kiwi Kale Gazpacho** (double batch); refrigerate in 1-cup portions. RECIPE PAGE 36	★ Make **Beet Soup with Fennel** (triple batch); refrigerate in 2-cup portions. RECIPE PAGE 58	**BREAKFAST** Apple & Amaranth Soup (2 cups)	★ Drink 2 cups of alkalized water between meals.
★ Make **Ancient Grains Soup** (triple batch); freeze in 2-cup portions. RECIPE PAGE 134	★ Make **Apple & Amaranth Soup** (double batch); refrigerate in 2-cup portions. RECIPE PAGE 100	★ Make **Bell Pepper Gazpacho** (triple batch); refrigerate in 2-cup portions. RECIPE PAGE 85	**SNACK** Beef & Poultry Bone Broth (2 cups) **LUNCH** Bell Pepper Gazpacho (2 cups)	★ Perform 30 to 60 minutes of light to moderate exercise daily during cleanse, particularly Pilates or yoga.
★ Eliminate processed foods and sugar from your diet and focus on whole foods.	★ Eliminate poultry, meat, and dairy from your diet. ★ Focus on vegetable-based meals supplemented with fish, grains, and legumes.	★ Transfer Beef & Poultry Bone Broth and Ancient Grains Soup from freezer to refrigerator to thaw. ★ Eliminate all animal products from your diet. ★ Eat vegetable-based meals with some legumes, grains, and nuts. ★ Drink at least 8 cups of water.	**SNACK** Beet Soup with Fennel (2 cups) **DINNER** Ancient Grains Soup (2 cups) **DESSERT** Kiwi Kale Gazpacho (1 cup) **ALTERNATIVES** Ginger Sweet Potato Soup (snack) RECIPE PAGE 96 Strawberry Rhubarb Soup (dessert) RECIPE PAGE 54	

The mix of onion, carrot, and celery that traditionally forms the base of many soups is called mirepoix.

VEGETABLE BROTH WITH BASIL

This **refreshing, light, and lemony** broth is the **perfect remedy** for cold season. For a **versatile vegetable soup base,** freeze a portion after straining and omit the **lemon and basil.** Serve hot.

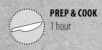

PREP & COOK
1 hour

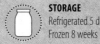

QUANTITY
Makes 8 cups
Serving size 2 cups

STORAGE
Refrigerated 5 days
Frozen 8 weeks

INGREDIENTS

1 TB. olive oil

1 cup celery, diced

1 cup carrot, peeled and diced

8 cloves garlic, whole

2 cups onion, diced

1 TB. black peppercorns, whole

6 stems parsley

8 cups purified water

1 bay leaf

Juice of 4 lemons

½ cup fresh basil, minced

½ tsp. salt

¼ tsp. pepper

METHOD

1 In a large stockpot, heat olive oil over medium heat for 2 minutes. Add onion, celery, carrot, and garlic. Cook until onion is translucent, about 5 minutes.

2 Add water, parsley, bay leaf, and peppercorns. Increase heat and bring to a boil, and then reduce heat, cover, and simmer for 40 minutes. Remove from heat.

3 Strain broth and discard vegetable solids. Stir in lemon juice and season with salt and pepper to taste. Let cool slightly before adding basil to prevent discoloration.

For an added...
metabolism boost, add very thinly sliced jalapeño or serrano pepper to broth.

NUTRITION PER SERVING

calories	17
total fat	0g
cholesterol	0mg
sodium	293mg
carbohydrate	6g
dietary fiber	1g
sugars	1g
protein	1g

CHILLED TOMATO CONSOMMÉ

This **light, chilled soup** captures the **essence of summer tomatoes**, highlighted with the **fresh herbal notes** of basil, tarragon, and chives. Enjoy as a **refreshing afternoon meal** or snack. Serve chilled.

 PREP & COOK
4 hours

QUANTITY
Makes 6 cups
Serving size 2 cups

STORAGE
Refrigerated 4 days
Frozen 8 weeks

INGREDIENTS

6 cups ripe tomatoes, quartered and cored

2 cups fennel, bulb and fronds, minced

2 cloves garlic, whole

2 cups onion, diced

2 tsp. sherry vinegar

2 TB. olive oil

2 TB. fresh basil, minced

1 TB. fresh tarragon, minced

1 TB. chives, thinly sliced

¼ tsp. salt

METHOD

1 In a blender or food processor, combine tomatoes, fennel, garlic, and onion. Purée until smooth.

2 Line a large, non-reactive bowl with a double layer of cheesecloth. Pour puréed vegetable mixture into the cloth, and then bring all four corners together and tie them to a wooden spoon. Place the spoon across the bowl so that the cheesecloth is hanging and contents can drip into bowl.

3 Transfer bowl with hanging cheesecloth to refrigerator and let sit for 4 to 6 hours or until the majority of the liquid has dripped through (it should yield about 6 cups). Discard cheesecloth and pulp.

4 Before serving, stir in sherry vinegar, olive oil, basil, tarragon, chives, and salt.

NUTRITION PER SERVING

calories	216
total fat	10g
cholesterol	0mg
sodium	248mg
carbohydrate	30g
dietary fiber	8g
sugars	16g
protein	6g

Experiment with... different herbs or even citrus flavors. Try dill and chive, or cilantro and lime zest.

For the greatest yield, use juicy tomato varieties with a high pulp content.

VUELVE A LA VIDA BROTH

Come back to life with this **spicy and restorative broth.** Warm, earthy cumin **boosts immunity** and **aids digestion,** while ground chiles clear congestion and **improve metabolism.** Serve hot.

 PREP & COOK
1 hour 10 minutes

QUANTITY
Makes 8 cups
Serving size 2 cups

STORAGE
Refrigerated 5 days
Frozen 8 weeks

INGREDIENTS

1 TB. olive oil

1½ cups onion, diced

1 cup carrot, peeled and diced

1 cup celery, diced

8 cloves garlic, whole

4 TB. tomato paste

8 cups purified water

5 stems parsley

1½ tsp. ancho chile powder

1 TB. ground cumin

¾ to 1½ tsp. chile de árbol

¼ tsp. salt

Juice of 4 limes

4 TB. cilantro, minced

METHOD

1 In a large stockpot, heat olive oil over medium heat for 2 minutes. Add onion, carrot, celery, and garlic. Cook until onion is translucent, about 5 minutes. Add tomato paste and cook for another 5 minutes.

2 Add water and parsley to pot. Increase heat and bring to a boil, and then reduce heat to simmer. Add ancho chile powder, cumin, and chile de árbol (adjust amount as desired). Cover and simmer for 40 minutes.

3 With a mesh seive or colander lined with cheesecloth, strain the broth, discarding vegetable solids. Season with salt and lime juice. Garnish with cilantro just before serving.

To make...
Tortilla Soup, add 1 cup canned fire-roasted tomatoes, 1 cup black beans, 1 sliced avocado, and a handful of crumbled tortilla chips.

NUTRITION PER SERVING	
calories	38
total fat	2g
cholesterol	0mg
sodium	88mg
carbohydrate	6g
dietary fiber	1g
sugars	2g
protein	2g

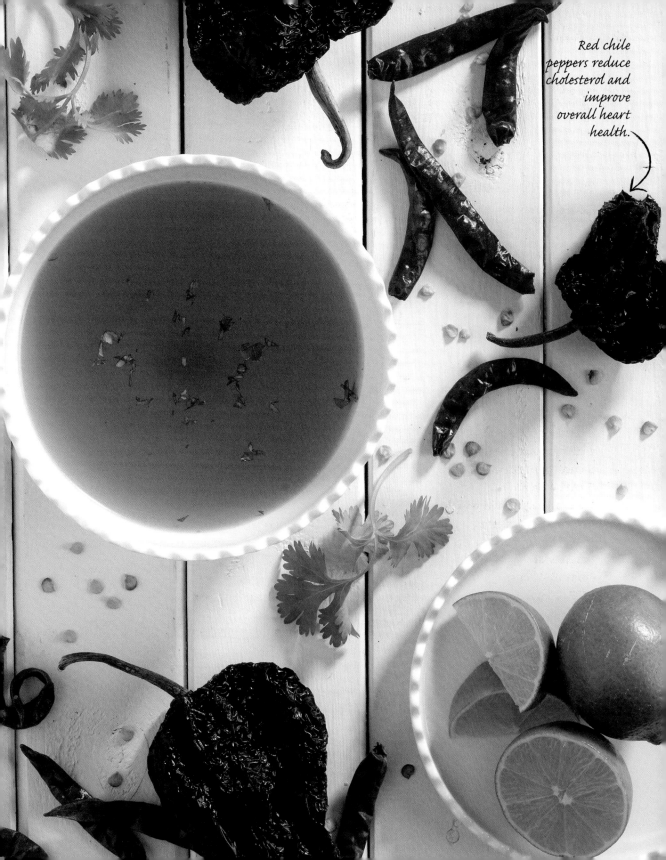

Red chile peppers reduce cholesterol and improve overall heart health.

Sweet corn is at its best at the end of summer. Make large batches of this broth and freeze to enjoy months later.

SWEET CORN BROTH

This **sweet and flavorful vegan broth** is perfect on its own or as a base for preparing **soups and cooked grains.** The broth is not only **mineral rich,** but also provides **vitamin C and folic acid.** Serve hot.

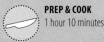 **PREP & COOK**
1 hour 10 minutes

 **QUANTITY**
Makes 6 cups
Serving size 2 cups

 **STORAGE**
Refrigerated 5 days
Frozen 8 weeks

INGREDIENTS

1 TB. coconut oil
½ cup celery, diced
½ cup onion, diced
6 ears sweet corn, kernels
  removed and cobs
  reserved
2 stems fresh thyme
2 stems fresh parsley
1 bay leaf
1 tsp. black peppercorns
8 cups purified water
¼ tsp. salt

METHOD

1 In a large stockpot, heat coconut oil over medium heat for 2 minutes. Add celery and onion and cook until vegetables are translucent, about 5 minutes.

2 Add corn kernels, corn cobs, thyme, parsley, bay leaf, black peppercorns, and water. Increase heat and bring to a boil, and then reduce heat, cover, and simmer for 40 minutes.

3 Strain to remove vegetable solids, leaving just the broth behind. Season with salt to taste.

Set aside...
1 cup of corn kernels and purée with the broth for increased dietary fiber and a thicker texture.

NUTRITION PER SERVING

calories	16
total fat	1g
cholesterol	0mg
sodium	99mg
carbohydrate	1g
dietary fiber	0g
sugars	0g
protein	0g

INDEX

ABOUT THE AUTHOR

Alison Velázquez is a wellness professional and founder of Soupology, a company specializing in innovative, health-focused soups. Soupology has been featured on the TODAY Show and is at the forefront of the new souping trend. With a background in both fitness and culinary arts, Alison has passion for healthy living that spans across all aspects of her life. A graduate of the School of Business at the University of Illinois,

Alison also received a certification in Pilates in 2009 and a Culinary Arts degree from Kendall College in Chicago. Having worked as both a private chef and caterer, she specializes in wellness cooking, utilizing fresh, seasonal ingredients to create light, unique fare. A vegetarian for nearly 20 years, Alison's specialty also lies in restricted dietary approaches, including vegan, Paleo, low carb, and gluten free.

ACKNOWLEDGMENTS

Credit is due to so many amazing supportive people who have helped shape and produce this unique cookbook.

Thanks to my family for teaching me the value of fresh quality ingredients, a deep appreciation for great food, and the value of a day's hard work.

To all of my friends and to Bug, thank you for your unwavering enthusiastic support; it's made all the difference.

A huge thank you to my clients for always supporting each of my new ventures and for having a genuine interest and commitment to healthy living that keeps me motivated and inspired to keep creating!

To all my Pilates people. You've been my reason to get out of bed every morning. Literally. Lucky for me, your commitment to your health and the latest gossip has been unwavering.

Thanks to Brook Farling, Ann Barton, and all those at DK who took a chance on me and made this whole project possible.

Thank you to Nigel Wright, Brian Wetzstein, and Mollie Hayward who brought my recipes to life through their beautiful photos and styling.

And a special thanks to Kimberley Watry for her wisdom and always lending an ear and a glass of wine for my countless quandaries.

PUBLISHER'S ACKNOWLEDGMENTS

The publisher would like to thank Maxine Pedliham—her trendspotting led to the publication of this book. Thanks are also due to Mary Rodavich, MS, RD, LDN for providing the nutritional analysis and to Carolyn Doyle for testing the recipes.